DATE DUE

MELTING POT

GARLAND REFERENCE LIBRARY
OF SOCIAL SCIENCE
(VOL. 351)

MELTING POT
*An Annotated Bibliography
and Guide to Food and Nutrition
Information for Ethnic Groups in America*

Jacqueline M. Newman, Ph.D., R.D.

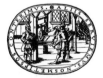

GARLAND PUBLISHING, INC. • NEW YORK & LONDON
1986

713158135
DLC

11-13-86ght

Library of Congress Cataloging-in-Publication Data

Newman, Jacqueline M., 1932–
    Melting pot.

do not use (Garland reference library of social science ;
vol. 351)
    Includes bibliographies.
    1. Food—Bibliography.   2. Diet—United States—
Bibliography.   3. Nutrition—Bibliography.   4. Food
habits—United States—Bibliography.   5. Cookery—
United States—Bibliography.   6. Ethnology—United
States—Bibliography.   I. Title.   II. Series: Garland
reference library of social science ; v. 351.
[DNLM: 1. Ethnic Groups—United States.   2. Food—
abstracts.   3. Nutrition—abstracts. ZQU 145 N553m]
Z7914.F63N48   1986   [TX353]   016.641   86-2140
ISBN 0-8240-4326-X

Cover design by Bonnie Goldsmith

Printed on acid-free, 250-year-life paper
Manufactured in the United States

Contents

ACKNOWLEDGMENTS

It is impossible to compile a volume such as this alone. There are, therefore, numerous people to whom I am in debt.

Thanks to my mother who opened my eyes to a multicolored world and my heart to allow entry. Thanks also to her friend, Professor Margaret A. Gram, who nudged my mind and body to learn, love, research, and teach in the field of home economics.

Thanks to the Interlibrary Loan Department of Queens College, CUNY, most particularly to Isabelle Taler and Ruth Hollander; without their efforts searching would have been both less pleasurable and less successful.

To my students, American and ethnic, and the many others too numerous to mention, whose cooperation raised my awareness, thanks to you, one and all.

Most important, I want to express my appreciation and love for my husband and best friend, whose moral support, cooperation, and perpetual concern aided my efforts and assured fruition.

PREFACE

This book addresses food, nutrition, and health related dietary concerns of the major ethnic groups in the United States. Through annotations it identifies cultural, social, and economic markers and provides knowledge of food habits, general dietary, nutriture, and related health problems and practices of the many ethnic groups that make up America's melting pot polyglot society.

Traditions and food habits vary from culture to culture. It is important to know, understand, and take into consideration ethnic beliefs and practices. To know and understand is to appreciate and help insure continuance of ethnic beliefs and practices that are meaningful and of value. To enable one to do so, this book offers help to those privileged to serve all the ethnics of America, be they colleagues, compatriots, friends, and/or neighbors.

The title of this volume does not propose or suppose that cultures melt. Rather, it considers that melting is the removal of barriers of misunderstanding, a means of appreciation and communication. This MELTING POT offers a way to study food in relation to all people and all people in relation to their food.

Before embarking on an armchair voyage of cultural understanding, I want to note the intent and limitations of the volume. It is my purpose to offer a wide variety of information specific to food and nutrition and related behavior in order to help the reader understand the varied populations groups.

The entries are but samples of many studies and published materials from diverse sources. They focus on the most recent ones and/or those that highlight particular ideas or issues. They were chosen to be representative and useful. They are not all inclusive. Their purpose is to enhance the reader's knowledge of ethnic groups.

It is inevitable that there be limitations. Errors of omission or commission may appear and are the sole responsibility of the author.

A Note on Format

The listings under "references" concentrate on general food habits, customs, behaviors, and nutrition related information about the particular ethnic group being discussed. The "resources for recipes" are lists of cookbooks that give advice on ingredients and preparation techniques, and more. Although often overlooked, cookbooks are excellent sources of food habits and food practices.

Inclusion of items is neither an endorsement nor a final word on a subject. Rather, inclusions are the author's suggestions of materials available from local libraries or through interlibrary loan. For more items consult the original sources and your local library.

This book is but an hors d'oeuvre in the repast of understanding. Knowledge about other cultures opens minds to appreciation and develops a sensitivity to the complexities of self and others. Read, learn, and enjoy, do so removing stones in the wall of ignorance about ethnics everywhere.

Melting Pot

Chapter 1

GENERAL INFORMATION

Ethnicity can be defined in many ways: for the purposes of this volume, it is the group or composite way that most people consider themselves, or the way outsiders think of them. That way or group can be nationality, region, and/or religion. These ways are not static because all cultures change. Among the changes are those expressed in food behaviors and cultural selection of foods whether made according to old and comforting or new and inviting ways.

Contemporary diets, the category of foods that are currently eaten, are based upon ethnic traditions. Many diets are rooted in ancient traditions that are of interest and value. These roots should be investigated. One tradition from ancient Chinese, Greek, and Hebrew literature indicates that when a person is ill the diet must be modified. If that does not effect a cure, then one should try medication. Another, from the same three ancient sources, indicates that grains with coats are healthy while too much meat is not. Old and new ideas affect food attitudes. They contribute to what people eat and why, just as ethnic and religious beliefs do.

America is a multi-ethnic place. Working and living in it one needs to understand people and be knowledgeable about the groups they represent. One way to become familiar with the major features of ethnic, regional, or religious food behaviors is to review the literature, investigate diet and disease patterns, and look at environmental and genetic factors that may contribute to them.

1.1   Food Habits: An Overview

Every culture has its own internal logic and coherence. Every culture is an intertwined system of values and attitudes of people with their own set of identities and food behaviors. Food selection is intricately tied up with culture. Early in life, patterns are established and set. To change is a difficult and slow process because habits develop and are based upon symbolic values, health perceptions, pleasant or unpleasant memories, and sensory or sensual exposures, all rooted in human experience. Food and food behaviors are not right or wrong, just different. They are different between individuals and between and within ethnic and cultural groups.

Man is unique among animals because he prepares and cooks his food. This culinary behavior is different in the varied cultures of man. Those who define themselves as belonging to a group, be they vegetarian or Vietnamese, interpret food preparation in individual, small group, and/or larger group terms bound by unique and individualized culinary practices. In people's decision making processes in selection and consumption of food, availability of the food itself, environmental variables, cost, social concerns, religious sanctions and taboos, palatability, ethnicity, and health benefits are all of concern.

Broad or specific acts of food behavior and salient choices and manipulations of food are how people mature, make their individual choices, and understand the choices and thereby the cultures of others. Other factors include immigration, acculturation, urbanization, and rapid social change; all are opportunities to take up new foodways or food habits. Radio, television, families with children in school, peers, work, convenience, and time saving are other influences as is the previously mentioned one of critical importance: ethnicity.

Ethnic food choices symbolize identification, they are important attachments to heritage. When circumstance, illness, or other health reasons require prudency or diet change, change can only be accommodated within the cultural context of what is known, liked, and valued. It can be difficult, even impossible, to attempt change outside an individual's culture and practice.

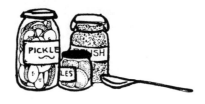

1.2 Ethnics in America

Over the past several hundred years, waves of immigrants have landed or touched down and spread across this nation seeking their fortunes. "Welcome to America" say the signs at dockside or international airports, and welcome the immigrants may feel as they move in with relatives and/or friends or start anew on their own in any of the fifty states.

Which are the states these waves of immigrants have moved to? One has only to read local or national newspapers and magazines to find out. For example, an ethnic map printed in 1979 in THE DAILY NEWS, a New York City newspaper, shows city residence concentrations at over 30 locations with dozens of ethnic groups there. Just six years later, TIME magazine, a national periodical, printed a map of the same city indicating that both areas and size of ethnic groups had more than tripled. That special July 8th issue showed immigrants altering the tastebuds of those in New York City and in cities and towns all over the United States. Miami, San Francisco, Chicago, Atlanta, Newark, and New Orleans are some of the cities that had increases of 25% or more in their foreign born populations.

Immigrants are continuing to change the face of America. They are adding many foods such as varieties of produce, breads, and seasonings. As they expand America's larder, Americans are naturalizing the foreign ingredients and recipes, calling them their own. In their turn the immigrants are acquainting themselves with America's foods.

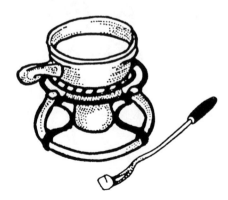

1.3   Who are the Immigrants?

The fastest growing group are Asians from China, the Philippines, Japan, India, South Korea, and Vietnam, with immigration up 133% in the years 1970 to 1980. Hispanics, the largest American minority, increased 61% in those same ten years. While northern and western Europeans arrived in droves at the beginning of the nineteenth century, change in the immigration acts during the 1960s caused the varieties and numbers of ethnics from other continents to swell. In the decade mentioned, the total minority population of the United States jumped from 17.1% to 20.5%.

Today about 50 million people are counted as minorities; numerous others remain uncounted. These new Americans are Asian, Hispanic, African, or European; White, Yellow, or Black; young, middle aged, or elderly; and rich, poor, or middle class. In 1980, with 87 maps and more than 1,000 pages, THE HARVARD ENCYCLOPEDIA OF ETHNIC GROUPS detailed who they are, where they live, and other information about 106 ethnic groups in America. The size of this volume reflects the magnitude of ethnics in America.

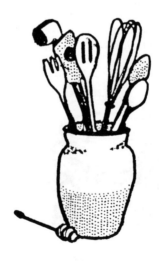

1.4 Who is Ethnic?

Ethnicity beyond the date of immigration and into second, third, and later generations is a matter of discussion, decision, and degree. No one, not those in the United States Census Bureau, not city planners, not politicians seeking votes can say for sure who consider themselves ethnics or where they live. What everyone does agree is that whatever called, ethnics or minorities, they are part of an ever growing polyglot population.

This mixed American population of minorities needs to be known and understood, their concerns and needs addressed by reading about them, listening to them, watching them, and appreciating their experiences. The need for knowledge and understanding is greatest in areas related to food, nutrition, and diet. Everyone has health concerns and eats several times a day. Everyone has health concerns that begin long before they are recognized.

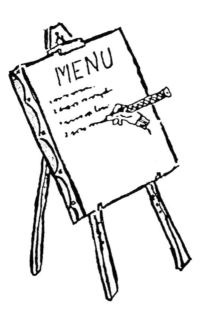

1.5   How Ethnic Populations Adapt

As immigrants partake of the land and its people, they use local foods, interpreting them in personal or traditional ways. No matter the influence, different nationals, different classes of people, and various religious groups have specific preferences and adapt their new knowledge to meet their own needs. The children of immigrants and the generations that follow continue to learn both the old ways and newer ways. They learn from radio, television, printed materials, overheard conversations, and from everyone and everything around them.

The chapters that follow are your way to learn. Use them to introduce yourself to the foods, nutrition, and related health concerns of different ethnic groups.

Chapter 2

BLACK AMERICANS

2.1 Introduction

Though grouped together in this chapter, it is important to point out that Black Americans are not one culture group and their food habits are not universal.

Black American food may be West Indian (see Hispanic), African, Southern United States soul food, or some other as the food habits of Black Americans reflect the region and/or the country that they and their ancestors came from. Though having traveled different paths, it is believed that all have common roots in Africa, a vast continent divided by the Sahara Desert, impenetrable jungles, and high mountains, a continent divided also by varied influences. Black American foods have, therefore, European, American, and indigenous African influences, predominantly the last. There are rural and urban differences, as well.

Cookery methods, more so than basic foods, distinguish regional and ethnic dishes of African origin. The African continent has had many influences, these are best generalized into major geographic sectors. North Africa is close to Middle Eastern food patterns. West Africa is based on tribal and Portuguese influences. South Africa was colonized by several countries, so the food habits are influenced by local tribes and those of the Dutch, French and English. East Africa, due to proximity and colonization, has English, Arab, and Indian influences.

People recently migrating from Africa have different food behaviors than do Black Americans here for generations. Among these recent immigrants, women are relagated to a subordinate role with regard to food habits. The men are given primary satisfaction at the dinner table; the women and children are frequently accorded the dregs of the meals and bear the brunt of traditional food taboos.

9

This is particularly true when the immigrant women remain at home and do not socialize.

Foods widely used as staples by Blacks of Africa and the Blacks of Central America are millet, corn, wheat, rice and barley, starchy roots and tubers such as cassavas and yams, plaintains and bananas, coconuts, ground nuts (peanuts), palm oil, kale, fish, and hot pepper-tomato-onion combinations in sauces and stews. Little meat is eaten and cooking styles are simple, often of the one-pot variety with starch. It is not uncommon for one cooked meal to be prepared and the rest of the day's food consumed only as snacks.

The principal staple food of many Blacks of Africa is often a starchy mixture. It is cooked with water and can be made from any cereal, tuber, starchy nut, or legume. It is often eaten with spicy sauces. This mixture can be soupy or prepared with less water, it can be fried or poached as are dumplings. Fruit wines, honey sweetened tea, coffee, and soft drinks are mealtime or between meal beverages.

Black Americans from the south of the United States and Blacks of other regional backgrounds have breakfast patterns similar to most other Americans. They also include grits in some form, and substitute biscuits, muffins, or corn-breads for yeast breads. At other meals, southern Blacks eat a good deal of okra, pidgeon peas, broad beans and collard, mustard, kale, and turnip greens. They like them long cooked and flavored with salt pork or fat back. When eating these greens, they consume the "pot likkor", as the cooking liquid is called. Other popular vegetables include sweet potatoes, squash, corn, and cabbage. Extensive use of pork and pork products and of offals are common to southern Black Americans as are hogs maw (stomach), chitterlings (intestines), and spare ribs. These and all foods, including grains, legumes, meats, poultry, and fish are preferred cooked with or fried in lard, barbecued, or stewed.

Most Black West Indians and others from Central America have Hispanic influences (which see) or influences of the European countries with whom their native country had past or present affiliation. An example of a non-Hispanic group would be the Haitians. They speak French and their food habits are influenced by them, and by Creoles and Indians.

For Blacks from Central and South American countries, fruits and vegetables are common dietary items while milk and most milk products including cheese are not used often. Buttermilk, evaporated milk, and ice cream are preferred dairy products but even these are not eaten in large amounts. Starchy vegetables are the bulk of the diet and meat and fish use is limited. Sweets are consumed frequently, particularly those flavored with molasses.

Religion also plays a part in food patterns. Some Black Americans are Seventh Day Adventists. Adventists in general are ovo-lacto-vegetarians. For them use of eggs, milk, and cheese are common; fish, and poultry are not. Meats, tea, coffee, and alcoholic beverages are forbidden foods. Diets of Seventh Day Adventists are similar to ovo-lacto-vegetarians but their starch consumption is high in tubers indigenous to their heritage countries.

Black American eating patterns share commonalities. Fried foods and sweetened flavored drinks are popular, smoked foods are, too. Breakfast used to be a large meal; it is now less so or light or non-existent. Snacks throughout the day and evening are very common, and currently, the evening meal is the largest of the day.

Depending upon their original roots, eating habits do differ but many Black Americans have diets consistently below the Recommended Dietary Allowances (RDA's) for energy, calcium, iron, vitamins C and A, and niacin. Dietary intake of sodium is high and related hypertension incidence is reported in several studies. This suggests that modifying intake may be beneficial. Sickle cell anemia, lower hematocrit levels, and high incidence of obesity have been reported along with hypertension and low intake of protein in some groups.

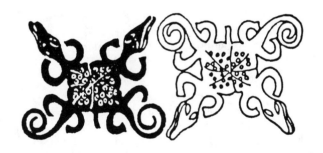

2.2 References

Bailey, F.E., and M.L. Walker. "Socio-economic factors and their effects on the nutrition and dietary habits of the Black aged." J. GERONTOL. NURS. 8,4 (1982): 203-207.

Selected literature examines socioeconomic status and nutrition of Black elderly. Evidence links health status and adverse dietary habits. Recommendations are: longitudinal studies to establish baseline data, counseling based on reality, social programs assuring financial resources, and information systems development.

Bailey, L.B., P.A. Wagner, C.G. Davis, and J.S. Dinning. "Food frequency related to folacin status in adolescents." J. AMER. DIETET. ASSOC. 84 (1984): 801-804.

Comparison of urban and rural households show urban Blacks select folacin dense foods more frequently than urban Hispanics or rural Blacks. Infrequent consumption of fruits and vegetables is one explanation of their poor folacin status.

Bailey, L.B., P.A. Wagner, G.J. Christakis, P.E. Araujo, H. Appledorf, C.G. Davis, J. Masteryanni, and J.S. Dinning. "Folacin and iron status and hematological findings in predominantly Black elderly persons from urban low-income households." AMER. J. CLIN. NUTR. 32 (1979): 2346-2353.

Sixty percent of the subjects classified as "high risk" have 140 ng/ml red blood cell folacin concentrations. Serum iron and transferrin saturation are normal or 15% for all subjects. Hematological indices show a 14% incidence of anemia with hemoglobin (12g/dl) and 32% incidence of leukopenia (leucocytes 4.8 x 10,000). Widespread folacin deficiency is demonstrated but there is no evidence of iron deficiency in the elderly studied.

Bailey, L.B., P.A. Wagner, G.J. Christakis, C.G. Davis, H. Appledorf, P.E. Araujo, E. Dorsey, and J.S. Dinning. "Folacin and iron status and hematological findings in Black and Spanish American adolescents from urban low-income households." AMER. J. CLIN. NUTR. 35 (1982): 1023-1032.

Folacin and iron status are low in both Black and Hispanic populations studied. Red blood cell folacin concentrations are less than 140 ng/ml in 42% of the 193 adolescents. The serum folacin values for 45% are below 6 ng/ml with levels decreasing with increasing age. Eleven percent of the females and 3% of the males are anemic with mean cell hemoglobin below 32% in 24% of the girls and 7% of the boys.

Blinkin, N.J., R.L. Williams, C.J.R. Hogue, and P.M. Chen. "Reducing Black neonatal mortality. Will improvement in birth weight be enough?" J. AMER. MED. ASSOC. 235 (1985): 372-378.

Comparison of California and Georgia neonates with weights under 3,000 gms. shows Blacks have lower mortality rates than Whites. In populations with birth weight over 3,000 gms., more Whites survive.

Bonham, G.S., and D.B. Brock. "The relationship of diabetes with race, sex, and obesity." AMER. J. CLIN. NUTR. 41 (1985): 776-783.

Data from 1976 National Health Interview Survey show 20.2% of the Blacks report diabetes; this is higher than disease incidence reported by Whites. Black men over age 65 are more obese than are Whites but the disease increases more rapidly among obese women than among men. There is no other consistent sex difference.

Bowering, J. "Infant nutrition in East Harlem." HUMAN ECOL. 6,4 (1976): 16-19.

Puerto Rican infants receive more homogenized whole milk than do Blacks in their first year of life though average nutrient differences show no differences in the formula or evaporated milk formula fed Black infants. Blacks introduce use of table foods earlier than do the Puerto Ricans.

Bowering, J., R.L. Lowenberg, and M.A. Morrison. "Nutritional studies of pregnant women in East Harlem." AMER. J. CLIN. NUTR. 33 (1980): 1987-1996.

Survey of 346 low-income pregnant women attending a clinic for high obstetric risk show about 25% had serum iron levels in the deficient range, about 20% had deficient plasma ascorbic acid levels, 7% had low red cell transketolase activity, 7% had marginal red cell riboflavin levels, and none had low plasma vitamin A levels. Women over age 35 ate less of many nutrients than did the teen-agers.

Brittin, H.C., and D.W. Zinn. "Meat buying practices of Caucasians, Mexican Americans and Negroes." J. AMER. DIETET. ASSOC. 71 (1977): 623-628.

Caucasian (C), Mexican American (M-A), and Negro (N) meat buying practices are observed in terms of kind of meat, weight, cost, and total money spent. Of more than 900 shoppers only 600 bought meat, and these were in 198 different cuts with only 33 types selected by more than 2% of the shoppers. Bacon was first choice of C's and M-A's, bologna and chicken second and third choices. N's chose chicken first, bacon second, and pork chops third. Ethnicity affected other purchases with N's households spending more money for pork, poultry, and fish than C's. Little fish was bought by any of the groups.

Cronin, F.J., S.M. Krebs-Smith, B.W. Wyse, and L. Light. "Characterizing food usage by demographic variables." J. AMER. DIETET. ASSOC. 81 (1982): 661-673.

Three-day food records of the 1977-78 USDA food intakes reveal age, race, and region affect percentage of persons using the 65 food groups and their mean frequency of use. Table shows these race differences.

Dickens, D., and R.N. Ford. "Food geophagy among Mississippi Negro school children." AMER. SOCIOL. REV. 7 (1942): 59-65.

Twenty-five percent of the boys and girls ate dirt during the 10- to 16-day interval investigated. Results are higher than other studies and were attributable to this study's hiding of critical and emotional words. No information given about the quantity consumed.

Dowd, J.J., and V.L. Bengtson. "Aging in minority populations." J. GERONTOL. 33 (1978): 427-436.

Black, Mexican American, and Whites of middle and older ages living in Los Angeles show life satisfaction or frequency of contact with relatives to be similar. Mexican American elderly show the greatest interaction with family and the least interaction with friends. Blacks and Mexican Americans were more likely to be in poor health and have low incomes than whites.

Driskell, J.A., A.J. Clark, T.L. Bazzarre, L.F. Chopin, H. McCoy, M.A. Kenney, and S.W. Moak. "Vitamin B-6 status of southern adolescent girls." J. AMER. DIETET. ASSOC. 85 (1985): 46-49.

Research addresses vitamin status using coenzyme stimulation of erythrocyte alanine aminotransferase and dietary intake of girls 12 to 16 years old. About half consumed less than 66% of the RDA's for this vitamin, 20% had marginal status, and 13% were deficient. Coenzyme stimulation and dietary values were similar for Whites and blacks in all age and income groups.

Farris, R.P., J.L. Cresanta, G.C. Frank, L.S. Weber, and G.S. Berenson. "Dietary studies of children from a biracial population: Intakes of carbohydrate and fiber in 10 and 13 year olds." J. AMER. COLLEGE NUTR. 4 (1985): 421-435.

Carbohydrate intake was similar for both sexes and Black and White races though boys consumed less sucrose and more lactose than did the girls. Starch, fiber, and glucose were higher in Black children with higher sucrose/starch intakes higher in White children. None of the children's intakes is compatible with prudent dietary recommendations of increased complex carbohydrate and decrease in use of simple carbohydrates.

Futrell, M.F., L.T. Kilgore, and F. Windham. "Nutritional status of Black pre-school children in Mississippi." J. AMER. DIETET. ASSOC. 66 (1975): 22-27.

Dietary interviewers ask the head of the household to record four days intake of his or her children's food. Height and weight are taken at the health center and dietary records checked for accuracy there. Boys have lower heights and weights compared to those in standard tables than do girls. Intake of nutrients from food and any supplements is low for iron, calcium, Vitamin A, and ascorbic acid regardless of income, education, sex, or food program participation.

Futrell, M.F., F. Windham, and L.T. Kilgore. "Hydroxyproline index: An indicator of nutritional status." J. AMER. DIETET. ASSOC. 67 (1975): 125-128.

Study evaluates 247 Black children's diet, height, weight, blood, and urine samples, and tests relationship between hydroxyproline and other indexes of nutritional status. Finds it has no advantage over height and weight as a nutrition status indicator.

Gardner, W.E. "The differential effects of race, education, and experience in helping." J. CLIN. PSYHCOL. 28 (1972): 87-89.

Study of 48 Black males and females seeing four Black and four White counselors found difference of race, experience, and education significant in counseling effectiveness; education was considered the least important.

Garn, S.M. "Lower hematocrit levels in Blacks are not due to diet or socioeconomic factors." PEDIATRICS 67 (1981): 580.

Editorial letter refutes diet and socioeconomic factors as causes of other differences between Blacks and Whites. Matched for income, food and iron intake, exercise, activity, and supplementation, hematocrit differences were real in the Ten State Nutrition Survey and other studies assessing more than 100,000 individuals.

Garn, S.M., A.S. Ryan, and S. Abraham. "The Black-White difference in hemoglobin levels after age, sex, and income matching." ECOL. FD. NUTR. 10 (1980): 69-70.

Black-White differences in hemoglobin approximate 0.72 gm, a value very close to that recorded for premenopausal women in study of 3,321 matched pair participants in the HANES I data set.

Garn, S.M., A.S. Ryan, G.M. Owen, and S. Abraham. "Income matched Black-White hemoglobin differences after correction for low transferrin saturations." AMER. J. CLIN. NUTR. 34 (1981): 1645-1647.

In 3,321 age-matched pairs from the HANES I survey, the magnitude of difference in hemoglobin approximates 0.73 gm/dl both before and after exclusion of low transferrin saturation levels.

Garn, S.M., H.A. Shaw, K.E. Guire, and K. McCabe. "Apportioning Black-White hemoglobin and hematocrit differences during pregnancy." AMER. J. CLIN. NUTR. 30 (1977): 461-462.

Editorial letter reports 17,825 pregnancy records with income corrections show that Black-White differences in hematocrit and hemoglobin levels do exist, with Blacks systematically lower in both. Analyses of variance place income-corrected Black-White differences close to 0.9g/100 ml for hemoglobin and close to 2.6% for the hematocrit.

Gillum, R.F. "Pathophysiology of hypertension in Blacks and Whites: A review of the basis of racial blood pressure differences." HYPERTENSION 1 (1979): 468-475.

Potential causes of hypertension include genetic factors, personal characteristics, renal physiology, endocrine factors, autonomic nervous system function, cardiac function, and various environmental factors. Extensive reference list.

Gladney, V.M. FOOD PRACTICES OF BLACK AMERICANS IN LOS ANGELES COUNTY. Los Angeles: County Department of Health Services, 1972.

Booklet includes summary of common food practices in the South and in Los Angeles County; shows high use of lard and pork products, limited use of milk and fruits, long cooking of greens, and large intake of soft drinks and candy. Instructions on how to evaluate dietary intake for Blacks, the questionnaire used in this study, and a summary of the practices of pre-school children are in the Appendix.

Grivetti, L.E. "Dietary separation of meat and milk a cultural-geographic inquiry." ECOL. FD. NUTR. 9 (1980): 203-217.

See under Middle Eastern References.

Haider, S.Q., and M. Wheeler. "Dietary intake of low socioeconomic Black and Hispanic teen-age girls." J. AMER. DIETET. ASSOC. 77 (1980): 677-681.

Study evaluates 150 teen-aged daughters of mother-daughter pairs in three groups by age: 13 to 14, 15 to 18, and 19 years old. Except for protein and ascorbic acid intake, which are higher than RDA's, intake of all nutrients either below or close to the RDA level. Iron intake is approximately 50% of RDA, calcium 33 to 78%, other nutrients near or below the RDA, and calories about 75% of the RDA's. Comparison of mothers and daughters show that nutrient intakes are not too different indicating similarity of meal patterns of both age groups. Ethnicity shows some differences: Black girls skip more meals and are slightly more obese than the Hispanic girls.

Haider, S.Q., and M. Wheeler. "Nutritive intake of Black and Hispanic mothers in a Brooklyn ghetto." J. AMER. DIETET. ASSOC. 75 (1979): 670-674.

Research of three-day dietary intake, food buying and preparation, and anthropometric analysis of 150 pairs of Black and Hispanic mothers and their teen-age daughters. Hispanics had better diets except for vitamin A and ascorbic acid nutriture. Both groups of mothers had low intakes of all nutrients except ascorbic acid, phosphorus, and protein. Low caloric intake of both ethnic groups, the prevalence of obesity, and high intake of protein indicate poor food choices and a need for nutrition education.

Haigh, N.Z., K.M. Salz, G.A. Chase, J.A. Jenkins, P.S. Bachorik, and P.O. Kwiterovitch. "The East Baltimore study: The relationship of lipids and lipoproteins to selected cardiovascular risk factors in an inner city Black adult population." AMER. J. CLIN. NUTR. (1983): 320-326.

Study of 24 males and 45 females shows compared to women, men consumed 9.3 more calories per kilogram of body weight, 273 mg. more cholesterol per day, and 7% fewer calories as sucrose. The P/S ratio of both their diets was 0.5. Mean lipid and lipoprotein levels were similar in men and women. The men's total cholesterol (167 mg/dl) and low density lipoprotein cholesterol (94 mg/dl) levels were lower than those of adult Blacks in other studies while the levels for women were similar to those of other studies.

Herring, B.D. "Cancer of the prostate in Blacks." J. NATL. MED. ASSOC. 69,3 (1977): 165-167.

Four areas showed that darker skin color was related to higher blood pressure independent of age, weight, socioeconomic status, etc. Findings suggested that varied gene mixtures, i.e., those with fathers from the West Indies might be related to blood pressure levels and that skin color, an indicator of possible metabolic significance, combined with socially induced stress to induce higher blood pressures in lower class Blacks. Companion article reviews Whites only.

Hein, K., M.J. Cohen, and H. McNamara. "Racial differences in nitrogen content of nails among adolescents." AMER. J. CLIN. NUTR. 30 (1977): 496-498.

Using the micro Kjeldahl technique, nail samples are analyzed in more than 150 adolescents in New York to assess body protein composition. There is a difference by race regardless of economic class or sex, with Blacks having 136 to 137 mg of nitrogen per nail while White values were 141 to 142 mgs. These value differences are significant and suggest that other indicators of protein synthesis need investigation.

Hill, P., L. Garbaczewski, P. Helman, J. Huskisson, E. Sporangisa, and E.J. Wynder. "Diet, lifestyle, and menstrual activity." AMER. J. CLIN. NUTR. 33 (1980): 1192-1198.

Lower levels of testosterone, androstenedione, dehydroepiandroesterone, and prolactin during the menstrual cycle were found in rural, Black South African women. When vegetarian Blacks ate a western diet, testosterone and prolactin levels rose. Western diet induced changes were comparable to those found in women with menstrual irregularities.

Hilliard, S.B. HOGMEAT AND HOECAKE: FOOD SUPPLY IN THE OLD SOUTH. Carbondale, IL: Southern Illinois University Press, 1972.

Provides considerable detail about food consumption in 1840-1860 concerning the roots of southern/soul food habits and diet as they existed in the antebellum era. Comments on nutritional aspects of the southern diet and food preferences of the people living there. Doctors' dietary recommendations are given, as are some references to twentieth-century dietary studies.

Hunt, I.F., H.M. Lieberman, A.H. Coulson, N.J. Murphy, and V.A. Clark. "Effect of a breakfast program on the nutrient intake of Black children." ECOL. FD. NUTR. 8 (1979): 21-36.

Comparison of children in schools with and without a breakfast program show mean intakes of both sets of children close to or greater than RDA's for all nutrients under study. Closer analysis reveals that 48% of the children report diets that provide less than two-thirds of the RDA for one or more nutrients. Differences between schools show that more children from the school without the breakfast program reported nothing eaten before 10 a.m.

Hunter, J.M. "Geophagy in Africa and the United States: A culture-nutrition hypothesis." GEOGRAPHICAL REV. 63 (1973): 170-175.

Study focuses on geophagy and physiological need. Analyses of Ghanian clays provide the basis for a culture-nutrition hypothesis using supporting and contrary research in previous studies. Geophagy in the United States, as a culture transfer from Africa, is discussed as are many studies of clay and starch eating.

Hunter, K.I., and M.W. Linn. "Cultural and sex differences in dietary patterns of the urban elderly." J. AMER. GERIAT. SOC. 27 (1979): 359-366.

Dietary patterns show Blacks more apt than Whites to rely on eggs and fatty meats and have overall negative meal ratings than do the Whites. Low socioeconomic status and education correlate positively with poor meal ratings.

Jackson, R.T., H.E. Sauberlich, J.H. Skala, M.J. Kretsch, and R.A. Nelson. "Comparison of hemoglobin values in Black and White male U.S. military personnel." J. NUTR. 113 (1983): 165-171.

Black men have 0.27 gm./dl lower mean hemoglobin values than do White men. In subjects with known iron intakes, about half of whom ate their meals in military dining facilities, the differences became smaller. The use of vitamin and mineral supplements are not significantly different between groups.

James, S.M. "When your patient is Black West Indian." AMER. J. NURS. 78 (1978): 1908-1909.

Knowledge of family stability, patterns of achievement, religious practices, and attitudes toward physical and mental work, and types of accustomed foods are all elements needed to provide effective and efficient care to this population.

Jerome, N.W. "Flavor preferences and food patterns óf selected U.S. and Caribbean Blacks." FOOD TECHNOL. (June 1975): 46-51.

Comparison of food patterns of Afro-Americans who grew up in the rural south and are now living in Wisconsin, with those of the Caribbean. Each transplanted population group has contemporary diet patterns based on traditional diets. Contemporary breakfast and dinner patterns of are shown with core, secondary core, and peripheral diet items. Traditional foods of the Caribbean islands are listed.

Jerome, N.W. FOOD HABITS AND ACCULTURATION: DIETARY PRACTICES AND NUTRITION OF FAMILIES HEADED BY SOUTHERN BORN NEGROES RESIDING IN A NORTHERN METROPOLIS. Ph.D. dissertation. University of Wisconsin, 1967.

Evidence of stability as well as change in diet exists. Vegetable consumption for good health remains an important value as does use of proper seasonings. Frozen vegetables when used are prepared according to package instructions, fresh are made by traditional means. Core of the diet remains traditional, foods high in ascorbic acid are generally not included. Change of attitudes and values in urban north are mostly from mass communication channels. Calcium and ascorbic acid are the limiting nutrients.

Jerome, N.W. "Northern urbanization and food consumption patterns of southern-born negroes." J. CLIN. NUTR. 22 (1965): 1667-1669.

Reviews dietary management and therapy by examining traditional, intermediate, and new meal patterns acquired during urbanization. Intermediate patterns show initial changes of diet in time and emphasis of meals. Urban new meal patterns indicate lighter breakfasts during the week, occupational lunches, and dinner as a combination of the traditional dinner and breakfast.

Johnson, C.C., and M.F. Futrell. "Anemia in Black preschool children in Mississippi." J. AMER. DIETET. ASSOC. 65 (1974): 536-541.

Indequate intakes of iron and folic acid are found in 150 pre-school Black children with 74% consuming less than 8 mg iron and 99% less than half the recommended allowance for folic acid.

Johnson, H.A. "The Afro-American in the melting pot." In ETHNIC AMER-
ICAN MINORITIES, edited by H.A. Johnson. New York: R.R. Bowker
Co., 1976.

Guide to media and materials begins with historical perspectives, social and
psychological needs of Afro-American youth entering mainstream America. Includes bibliography on these topics, annotated information on films, filmstrips,
slides, audio and video cassettes, and some graphics materials.

Kafatos, A.G., and P. Zee. "Nutritional benefits from federal assistance."
AMER. J. DIS. CHILD. 131,3 (1977): 265-269.

Studies 250 of approximately 4,000 pre-school Black children whose families
participated in one or more federal programs and shows improvements in height
and weight and reduction in numbers of children with anemia and low plasma
vitamin A levels.

Kilcoyne, M.M., G.E. Thomson, G. Branche, M. Williams, C. Garnier, B.
Chiles, and T. Soland. "Characteristics of hypertension in the Black
population." CIRCULATION 50 (1974): 1006-1013.

Examines 146 Black patients with hypertension and finds low renin and reduced sodium excretion as measured by radio-immunoassay of Angiotensis I and
the accompanying sodium excretion. Suggests incidence of vascular events may
relate to more angiotension-vascular receptor interaction than to measurement
of circulating renin.

King, M.H., F.M.A. King, D.C. Morley, H.J.L. Burgess, and A.P. Burgess.
NUTRITION FOR DEVELOPING COUNTRIES. London and Nairobi:
Oxford University Press, 1972.

Materials throughout make reference to maize, cassava, and millet areas of
Africa. Most examples are taken from Zambia but they are applicable in other
countries. Though the book is intended as a nutrition text for use in Africa,
the materials about meeting dietary needs, adjusting to customs and culture,
and helping families and community to help themselves are useful for similar
populations worldwide.

Kliman, D.S. "Racial preferences expressed for peers and adults by preschool
children." HOME ECON. RES. J. 5,3 (1977): 143-145.

Results of 24 pairs of Black and White children show favorable perceptions
by Blacks for others of like skin color. Implications are for selection of adult role
models.

Koh, E.T. NUTRITION SURVEY OF BLACK FAMILIES IN CLAIBORNE
   COUNTY OF SOUTHWEST MISSISSIPPI: II. HEALTH HISTORI-
   CAL, CLINICAL AND ANTHROPOMETRIC FINDINGS, 1976. Lor-
   man, MI: Alcorn State University, 1978.

Study details 200 Black families where anemia is prevalent in all age categories, though more among females and the elderly. Asthma is found in children
under 12 and females over 34, hayfever reported in 25% of those over 35. Males
aged 18-34 have the highest rate of allergic reactions, goiter is a problem only
with females over age 17, diabetes prevalent in older females, more obesity in
the old than in the young, and more in females than males. Clinical findings
indicate higher prevalence of nutrient deficiency than did subjects in the HANES
study except for vitamin C and protein.

Koh, E.T. "Selected anthropometric measurements for a low-income Black
   population in Mississippi." J. AMER. DIETET. ASSOC. 79 (1981): 555-
   561.

Study of 200 Black households shows all anthropometric measurements increase with age. Blood pressure and skinfold thickness are greater in female
subjects while males are always taller at a comparable age. Hypertension is
more prevalent among females as is obesity.

Koh, E.T. "Selected blood components and urinary B as related to age and
   sex of a Black population in Southwest Missouri." AMER. J. CLIN.
   NUTR. 33 (1980): 670-676.

Results of study of 200 households indicate that blood components and urinary B vitamins are affected by age and sex. While hematocrit, White blood
cells, globulin, glucose, and cholesterol significantly increase with age, vitamin
C, and urinary thiamin values consistently decrease. Red blood cells, calcium,
and albumin values are independent of age. Hematocrit, hemoglobin, and serum
iron levels are significantly higher in males.

Koh, E.T., and S.C. Myung. "Clinical signs found in association with nutritional deficiencies as related to race, sex, and age for adults." AMER. J.
   CLIN. NUTR. 34 (1981): 1562-1568.

Clinical signs of deficiency are much higher for vitamin A, riboflavin, vitamins C and D, and calcium in the 429 adults of this study. Men showed higher
prevalence than did women of clinical signs of deficiency of all nutrients. Older
people did likewise, except for vitamin A. In comparison with the HANES data,

1971 to 1974, White subjects had slightly higher clinical signs of deficiency while Blacks had still higher.

Koh, E.T., S.C. Myung, and F.W. Lowenstein. "Comparison of selected blood components by race, sex, and age." AMER. J. CLIN. NUTR. 33 (1980): 1828-1835.

Study observes a significant racial difference for 429 Black and White adults in southwest Mississippi except for alpha-1-globulin, cholesterol, and alkaline phosphatase. Albumin, apha-2-globulin, hemoglobin, hematacrit, serum iron, triglycerides, and vitamin C are significantly higher in Whites than in Blacks and total protein, beta-1 and gamma-globulins, and glucose are significantly higher in Blacks. Those 60 and over have higher gamma-globulin and alkaline phosphatase, while adults under 60 have higher hematocrits.

Latham, M. HUMAN NUTRITION IN TROPICAL AFRICA. Rome, Italy: Food and Agriculture Organization of the United Nations, 1965.

Textbook for health workers addresses community health problems in East Africa with sections on public health, malnutrition, foods, practical solutions to nutrition problems, and diets for various ages and institutions. Insights useful worldwide.

Lee, C.J. "Nutritional status of selected teenagers in Kentucky." AMER. J. CLIN. NUTR. 31: (1978): 1453-1464.

Nutrition survey of 118 boys and girls ages 12 to 19 shows boys have higher intakes in overall nutrients and more regular meal habits than do girls. Intakes of calcium, iron, and vitamin A are grossly deficient in Black and White girls, and there is a high incidence of obesity among this group. Black boys have higher blood pressures. Blacks of both sexes show elevated serum cholesterol, beta-lipoprotein levels, and are less physically active than are Whites.

Leung, W.T.W. A SELECTED BIBLIOGRAPHY ON AFRICAN FOODS AND NUTRITION AND AFRICAN BOTANICAL NOMENCLATURE. Rome, Italy: Office of International Research of the NIH and Consumption and Planning Branch of the FAO, 1976.

Lists and annotates food habits, food composition, nutrition, and botanical literature on foods and diets in Africa.

Liebman, M., M.A. Kenney, W. Billon, A.J. Clark, G.W. Disney, E.G. Ercanli, E. Glover, H. Lewis, S.W. Moak, J.H. McCoy, P. Schilling, F. Thye, and T. Wakefield. "Iron status of Black and White female adolescents from eight Southern states." AMER. J. CLIN. NUTR. 38 (1983): 109-114.

Black females ages 12, 14, or 16 had significantly lower mean hemoglobin, hematocrit, and transferrin saturation levels than did Whites. Adjusting for dietary iron intakes and per capita income levels did not adequately account for the significant race differences for iron status parameters in the 1,000 girls studied.

Luft, F.C., C.E. Grim, J.T. Higgins, and M.H. Weinberger. "Differences in response to sodium administration in normotensive White and Black subjects." J. LAB. CLIN. MED. 90 (1977): 555-562.

Sixty-eight matched pair White and Black subjects infused with two liters of normal saline solution to elevate suppression of the renin-aldosterone system have similar responses to normal saline and furosemide administration. Blacks excrete significantly less sodium and potassium than Whites and their plasma renin activity is significantly suppressed, as well.

McCabe, K. "Apportioning Black-White hemoglobin and hematocrit differences during pregnancy." AMER. J. CLIN. NUTR. 30 (1977): 461-462.

Evaluating large numbers of Black-White differences, letter to the editor suggests that most of the 17% variance in hemoglobin in pregnant women is attributable to race, with only 1% to income. New data involving hemoglobin and hematocrit during pregnancy place income-corrected difference close to 0.9g/100ml for hemoglobin and close to 2.6% for hematocrit. Great differences in all ages and both sexes suggest race specific norms appropriate.

McCoy, H., M.A. Kenney, A. Kirbey, G. Disney, F.G. Ercanli, E. Glover, M. Korsland, H. Lewis, M. Liebman, E. Livant, S. Moak, S.F. Stallings, T. Wakefield, P. Schilling, and S.J. Ritchey. "Nutrient intakes of female adolescents from eight southern states." AMER. J. DIETET. ASSOC. 84 (1984): 1453-1460.

Nutrients calculated from two 24-hour recalls of more than 1,200 adolescent Black and White females indicate that Whites consume more vitamins C, D, E, and B-12, niacin, folacin, calcium, phosphorus, magnesium, iron, zinc, and protein, than do Blacks. Urban respondents consume more calories and magnesium than rural females and folacin intake increases with income. The majority of diets met or exceeded RDA's for protein, vitamins C, E, B_{12}, riboflavin, and thiamin.

McLoughlin, P.F.M. AFRICAN FOOD PRODUCTION SYSTEMS – CASES AND THEORY. Baltimore: Johns Hopkins University Press, 1970.

Text focuses on food problems in seven African societies and gives daily schedule of its people, frequently mentioning foods consumed, kinship relationships, and general behaviors.

Marrs, D.C. "Milk drinking by the elderly of three races." J. AMER. DIETET. ASSOC. 72 (1978): 495-498.

Eighty-five percent of the Mexican Americans, 93.5% of the Blacks, and 94% of the Whites who are not Mexican American reported drinking milk at meals at a Title VII program in Texas. Only 6.6%, 1.4%, and 2.5% of the respective groups do not consume milk because of intolerance symptoms. Buttermilk is preferred by 4%, 22%, and 16% of these groups, respectively.

May, J. THE ECOLOGY OF MALNUTRITION IN MIDDLE AFRICA. New York: Hafner Publishing Co., 1965.

Fifth volume in Medical Geography series, the first on Africa. Focuses on Ghana, Nigeria, the Congo, and former French Equatorial Africa (including Gabon, Congo, Central African Republic, and Chad). Each section details background, food resources, diet, adequacy of food, and nutritional disease patterns, has concluding remarks and bibliography, tables and maps about the country. This research is sponsored by Natick Laboratories, U.S. Army. It includes extensive bibliographic references.

May, J. THE ECOLOGY OF MALNUTRITION IN NORTHERN AFRICA. New York: Hafner Publishing Co., 1967.

Volume seven of this series, the second on Africa includes Libya, Tunisia, Algeria, Morocco, Spanish Sahara and Infi, and Mauritania. Format is the same as above.

May, J. THE ECOLOGY OF MALNUTRITION IN THE FRENCH SPEAKING COUNTRIES OF WEST AFRICA AND MADAGASCAR. New York: Hafner Publishing Co., 1968.

Volume eight of this series includes Senegal, Guinea, Ivory Coast, Togo, Dahomey, Cameroon, Niger, Mali, Upper Volya, and Madagascar. Format is the same as detailed above.

May, J. THE ECOLOGY OF MALNUTRITION IN EASTERN AND FOUR COUNTRIES OF WESTERN AFRICA. New York: Hafner Publishing Co., 1970.

Volume nine in this series includes Equatorial Guinea, Gambia, Liberia, Sierra Leone, Malawi, Zambia, Rhodesia, Kenya, Tanzania, Uganda, Ethiopia, Territory of Afars and Issas, Somali, and the Sudan. The format is the same as detailed above.

May, J.M., and D.L. McLellan. THE ECOLOGY OF MALNUTRITION IN SEVEN COUNTRIES OF SOUTHERN AFRICA AND IN PORTUGUESE GUINEA. New York: Hafner Publishing Co., 1971.

The last volume in the series on Africa includes South Africa, Namibia, Botswana, Lesotho, Swaziland, Mozambique, Angola, and Portuguese Guinea. Format is as detailed above.

Medeiros, D.M., and R.F. Borgman. "Blood pressure in South Carolina children." J. ROYAL SOC. HEALTH. 104 (1984): 68-71.

Modest differences in blood pressure are noted for Black and White children with a trend to lower blood pressure in both Blacks and Whites when breakfast is eaten regularly.

Morrison, J.A., I. deGroot, K.A. Kelly, M.J. Mellies, P. Khoury, B.K. Edwards, D. Lewis, A. Lewis, M. Fiorelli, G. Heiss, H.A. Tyroler, and C.J. Gleuck. "Black-White differences in plasma lipids and lipoproteins in adults: The Cincinnati lipid research clinic population study." PREV. MED. 8 (1979): 34-39.

Black males in 43 matched pair groups show lower plasma triglycerides and higher plasma high density lipoprotein cholesterol than do Whites. The ratio of low density to high is lower in Black males with no differences in females. Black females have slightly lower plasma triglycerides and slightly higher high density lipoprotein cholesterol than White females.

Parker, S.L., and J. Bowering. "Folacin in diets of Puerto Rican and Black women in relation to food practices." J. NUTR. EDUC. 8 (1976): 73-76.

Folacin content of diets of both groups appear adequate. Little folacin loss occurs from kidney beans after cooking. Other food preparation methods are conducive to folacin retention yet these populations have high incidence of megaloblastic anemia. Food habit modifications given to achieve higher folacin intake.

Reeves, J.D., D.A. Driggers, E.Y.T. Lo, and P.R. Dallman. "Screening for anemia in infants: Evidence in favor of using identical hemoglobin criteria for Blacks and Caucasians." AMER. J. CLIN. NUTR. 34 (1981): 2154-2157.

In year-old infants, 37% of the Blacks and 22% of the Caucasians have hemoglobin values below 11.5 gm/dl. When treated with oral iron for three months, the percentage increase in hemoglobin value is similar for both races.

Schuck, C., and J.B. Tartt. "Food consumption of low-income, rural Negro households in Mississippi." J. AMER. DIETET. ASSOC. 62 (1973): 151-155.

Records of 461 households reveal very low incomes, education of females higher than males, meat and grains contributing most of the calories, and about one-half of the fat calories from meats.

Segall, M.H. CROSS-CULTURAL RESEARCH IN NUTRITION. Syracuse, NY: Program of East African Studies of Maxwell Graduate School of Citizenship and Public Affairs, 1970.

Synopsis and research guide emphasizes Eastern Africa and discusses malnutrition's psychological effects, particularly on children. This longitudinal study will assess dozens of behavioral measurements, household food surveys, related food habit information, and socioeconomic indicators. Methodology is discussed as a model; the research is still in progress.

Segall, M., and P. Ulin, editors. TRADITIONAL HEALTH CARE DELIVERY IN CONTEMPORARY AFRICA. Syracuse, NY: African Series of the Maxwell School, n.d.

Analysis of the medical practices in modern Africa with considerable emphasis on ethnomedical beliefs, traditional healing and curing, and the impact of modern medical practices.

Sexton, D.E. "Black buyer behavior." J. MARKETING 36 (1972): 36-39.

Study indicates that income explains many behavioral buying differences between Blacks and Whites. Convenience of store location and friendly atmosphere outweigh price as Blacks spend proportionally more than Whites for food and medical care.

Siegel, J.M. "A brief review of the effects of race in clinical service interactions." AMER. J. ORTHOPSYCHIAT. 44 (1974): 555-562.

Literature concerning Black patient and White clinician indicates race shows little empirical differences in treatment success. One exception is that Black patients should be paired with Black staff for the intake interview.

Sloane, B.A., C. Gibbons, and M. Hegsted. "Evaluation of zinc and copper nutritional status and effects upon growth of southern adolescent females." AMER. J. CLIN. NUTR. 42 (1985): 234-241.

Biracial sample of 29 fourteen-year-old and 30 sixteen-year-old females indicates plasma zinc differences are significantly lower for Blacks. Mean plasma copper was slightly higher for Blacks than Whites. Plasma copper levels are related to size.

Stephenson, L.S., M.C. Latham, and D.V. Jones. "Milk consumption by Black and by White pupils in two primary schools." J. AMER. DIETET. ASSOC. 71 (1977): 258-262.

Study reports that in 222 primary school children in Ithaca, New York, race alone does not affect milk consumption at school or home. Abdominal pain or discomfort not reported, though more than 200 drank an average of three glasses a day and have other sources of dairy products in their diets.

Vilhjalmsdottir, L., A.G. Ferris, V.A. Beal, and P.L. Pellet. "Short stature and overweight in infants of western Massachusetts." ECOL. FD. NUTR. 8 (1979): 127-135.

Study of 268 urban Black, White, and Puerto Rican infants age one to 26 weeks and from three economic levels indicates that girls from low income families tend to be heavier, low income Black children are longer, and all girls are generally less heavy than boys in the same height group.

Voors, A.W., E.R. Dalferes, Jr., G.C. Frank, G.G. Aristimuno, and G.S. Berenson. "Relation between ingested potassium and sodium balance in young Blacks and Whites." AMER. J. CLIN. Nutr. 37 (1983): 583-594.

Black and White normotensive volunteers took 80mEq. potassium chloride daily in addition to their regular diets. Urine and stool samples for three days show Black children had negative sodium balance and a more positive cumulative potassium balance than did White children. Dietary enrichment affects their sodium balance.

Wagner, P.A., M.L. Krista, L.B. Bailey, G.J. Christakis, J.A. Jernigan, P.E. Araujo, H. Appledorf, C.G. Davis, and J.J. Dinning. "Zinc status of elderly Black Americans from urban low-income households." AMER. J. CLIN. NUTR. 33 (1980): 1771-1777.

Zinc content of hair and serum of 135 elderly Black, aged 60 to 87, suggests that the zinc status may be less than ideal though lesions sometimes associated with zinc deficiencies were not observed in any of the subjects. Hair zinc concentrations are not significantly lower in those 33 individuals reporting use of antihypertensive agents and/or cardiotonic medications.

Wheeler, M., and S.Q. Haider. "Buying and food patterns of Ghetto Blacks and Hispanics in Brooklyn." J. AMER. DIETET. ASSOC. 75 (1979): 560-563.

Study surveys mothers to learn their patterns of food management. All are of low income and over half have lived in New York at least 19 years. Most rank budgeting their number one problem. Black mothers rank planning second, and shopping third, Hispanic mothers reverse these. Both groups fry foods most and broil least. Similarities of mothers are greater than differences; education, except for language, could be planned in the same manner for both.

Williams, D.A. "Racial differences of hemoglobin concentration: Measurement of iron, copper, and zinc." AMER. J. CLIN. NUTR. 34 (1981): 1694-1700.

Mean hemoglobin of Black males is 0.9gm/dl less than that of White males and 0.5gm/dl less than that of White females. Differences cannot be explained by iron, copper, or zinc nutriture. Ferratin values of White females are significantly lower than those observed in White males but not in the Black population of this study. Red blood cells of all Blacks are smaller than those of Whites.

Williams, R.A., editor. TEXTBOOK OF BLACK-RELATED DISEASES. New York: McGraw-Hill Book Co., 1975.

Twenty chapters, each by experts in their own fields detail gap in health status between Black and White Americans, genetics and Black diseases, obstetrics and gynecology, pediatrics, hematology, endocrine diseases, hypertension, cardiology, pulmonary disease, infectious diseases, dermatology and venereology, neurology, digestive diseases and malnutrition, alcoholism, drug abuse, psychiatric states, Black suicide, voodoo medicine, surgery and oncology, and opthamology. Detailed references are given after each chapter and include many research studies. Current medicines are given with dosages included where appropriate. The chapter on voodoo medicine is of interest as it charts illness, remedy, ingredients and/or preparation, and how the substances are given.

Wyant, K.W., and H.L. Meiselman. "Sex and race differences in food preferences of military personnel." J. AMER. DIETET. ASSOC. 84 (1984): 169-175.

Preference ratings show orange juice and milk preferred by Black and White men and White women. Blacks prefer and select fruit and fruit juices most often and women of both races prefer vegetables, salads, and fruit more than men.

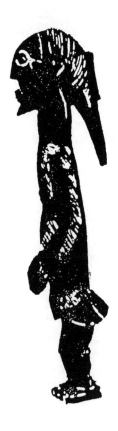

2.3   Resources for Recipes

Bailey, M. BLACK AFRICA COOK BOOK. San Francisco: Determined
Productions, 1977.

Some recipes in this paperback indicate they are from Ethiopia, Uganda,
Tanzania, Ghana, or Senegal; most do not. All are Americanized but with the
taste of Black Africa.

Burgess, M.K. SOUL TO SOUL, A VEGETARIAN SOUL FOOD COOK-
BOOK. Santa Barbara, CA: Woodbridge Press, 1975.

Recipes for all courses have soul flavor and no meat. Casseroles and entrees
use vegeburger, its recipe included, gluten steaks, TVP, soyameats, other meat
substitutes, and/or meat style seasonings. Fried chicken, pepper steak, and corn
dog recipes central to soul cookery, are made from vegetables.

Coetzee, R. THE SOUTH AFRICAN CULINARY TRADITION. Capetown,
South Africa: C. Struik, Publishers, 1977.

Author traces the interrelation of cultural background, eating habits, and
social practices in the early Cape Dutch community from 1652 to 1800. Text is
well researched and accompanied by 167 authentic recipes, most still used today.
Illustrations from museums or museum items set the dishes in period displays.
Recipes in metric and non-metric measures for use in America. Though written
with the flavor of earlier times, can be reproduced today.

Hatchen, H. KITCHEN SAFARI. New York: Atheneum, 1970.

Recipe chapters are divided by North, West, Southern, Central and East
Africa. Throughout, the author intersperses travelog with recipes. A glossary
of African food terms and list of recommended substitutions included.

Jackson, R. RUTH JACKSON'S SOULFOOD COOKBOOK. Memphis, TN:
Wimmer Books, 1978.

Thirteen typical soul food dishes begin this book of southern and soul cooking
chapters follow, desserts the largest recipe section.

Kaiser, I.Y. SOUL FOOD COOKERY. New York: Pitman Publishing Co.,
1968.

Southern Black recipes include beverages through desserts. Assorted tips on
saving time, money, and using leftovers.

Koeune, E. COOKING FOR THE FAMILY IN EAST AFRICA. Kampala:
    East African Literature Bureau, 1974.

Written for cookery teachers in the schools of the region, the book discusses
kitchens, equipment, sanitation, preservation, storage, planning and cookery
methods, menus, food for invalids, advice, hints, and recipes.

Lewis, E.L. TASTE OF COUNTRY COOKING. New York: Alfred A. Knopf,
    1976.

In recipes and reminiscences, the author shares the country cooking of Vir-
ginia she grew up with. The book is divided into four seasonal sections, Spring,
Summer, Fall, and Winter, with recipes that are southern and soul style. They
are presented as breakfast, lunch and dinner menus.

McQueen, A.B., and A.L. McQueen. WEST AFRICAN COOKING FOR
    BLACK AMERICAN FAMILIES. New York: Vantage Press, 1982.

Included are West African recipes from appetizers through desserts, a food
glossary, and a list of ingredient substitutes.

Odarty, B.A. SAFARI OF AFRICAN COOKING. Detroit: Broadside Press,
    1971.

Fact sheet of name of country, its capital, date of independence, former
sovereignty, area, population at press time, a map of Africa, and recipes, most
of them collected from the embassies begins each national section after a short
paragraph about the land, people, and their respective food habits.

Pamela, P. PRINCESS PAMELA'S SOUL FOOD COOKBOOK. New York:
    New American Library, 1969.

Afro-American recipes, part southern and part soul style, are divided into
five sections entitled: Meats complete 'n other soul treats; Sweet garden greens,
roots 'n shoots; Grits, 'taters, rice 'n mush; Batter 'n butter; and Soulfood
goodies. Poems about people and culture are on pages on the left, recipes on
the pages on the right.

Sandler, B. THE AFRICAN COOKBOOK. New York: World Publishing
    Co., 1970.

Menus and details of presentation are from 11 countries, Ethiopia, The Sudan, Morocco, Senegal, Kenya, Tanzania, Mozambique, Malagasy, South Africa,
Liberia and Ghana, and the Island of Zanzibar. An African buffet, additional

recipes categorized from appetizers to beverages, food habits, and culinary and cultural items also detailed.

Tuesday Magazine, editor. THE TUESDAY SOUL FOOD COOKBOOK. New York: Bantam Books, 1969.

Southern recipes billed as "America's soul food favorites" first appeared in the magazine; they are divided into meal courses from bread through beverages.

van der Post, L., editor. AFRICAN COOKING. New York: Time-Life Books, 1970.

Chapters on Ethiopia, East Africa, Portuguese Africa, the area at the Cape. Places throughout the continent are discussed from the personal perspective of the author. Recipes give country of origin. Book accompanied by one titled RECIPES; AFRICAN COOKING which includes only the recipes, no textual materials.

Wilson, E.G. A WEST AFRICAN COOKBOOK. New York: Avon Books, 1971.

Foods adapted for American kitchens are from Ghana, Liberia, Nigeria, and Sierra Leone. Chapters praise pepper, detail other characteristics of West African food, clarify ingredients, and advise on cooking and eating the West African way. There are other culinary and cultural items, feasts and rituals, and a recommended list of regional cookbooks and food articles.

Chapter 3

HISPANIC AMERICANS

3.1 Introduction

The United States has the sixth largest Spanish-speaking population in the world exceeded only by Mexico, Spain, Colombia, Argentina, and Peru. In recent years there has been a dramatic increase in this population, often referred to as Hispanic.

No universal definition exists of the term Hispanic, often it has been used to describe those people who trace their origin or descent to the Spanish-speaking areas of the Caribbean or Central or South America. Not everyone agrees with this definition, however; those who consider themselves Hispanic and those who define them as such may be referring to different population groups. In the United States there is a heterogeneous group of people from 21 Spanish-speaking countries, having different diets, habits, customs, and cultures; some of these people may consider themselves Hispanic, some not.

Hispanic people are classified by the United States Census Bureau as an ethnic not a racial group, though in the census data some Hispanics are presumed to have reported themselves as White or Black and not Hispanic. Therefore, data on this population and on the Black population may not be accurate.

Close to one million Hispanics, who reported themselves as such to census takers, lived in New York City in 1970. In 1980, the Hispanic population in New York City and the Hispanic population in the nation more than doubled, the latter to approximately 17 million. It is thought that three or more million were unaccounted for because they are immigrants without legal status. The Hispanic population in the United States is projected to reach 40 million by 1990.

Hispanic-American cuisines and cultures are diverse because of the influences

35

of European countries such as France, Holland, Denmark, England, Spain, Portugal, as well as many countries of North and South America and Africa. Length of residence in the United States affects the food habits of Hispanic-Americans. Some, like the Puerto Ricans, have a large population that has been here for many generations, while others, like those from Cuba and El Salvador, have had dramatic increases in their populations in recent years.

The Hispanic population in the United States is thought to be 60% Mexican, 15% Puerto Rican, 7% Cuban, and the rest mostly Central and South American. No matter what the numbers, some generalities do emerge, and in food habits and customs these include the large use of beans, rice, and bananas as diet staples. Foods and spices that are less used but still popular include avocados, mangoes, cilantro, garlic, and red apples. Most Hispanics eat some fish, dried or fresh, more poultry, some milk and fruit juices, and some kinds of cheese. Frozen food is becoming popular among Hispanics, especially the use of fried potatoes, pizza, and orange juice. If rice and beans were available frozen, they would be well accepted.

3.1.1   Mexican Americans

The people from Mexico are often referred to as Chicanos though the term can refer to Central Americans as well. The diet of Mexican Americans differs from one locale to another and is based upon Indian and Spanish influences. Typical foods are dried beans, chili peppers, and corn. Meat, fish, poultry, and eggs are eaten, but only if affordable. Meats are enjoyed marinated or well seasoned, ground or cut in pieces. They are used in many ways: in the sausage called chorizo, in empanadas, piccadillos, burritos, and tostados. These protein foods supplement legumes of all kinds, including black, garbanzo, kidney, or pinto beans. They are served alone or mixed with rice.

Dairy product intake is limited; dairy products are used primarily in flan (baked custard), mild cheeses, ice cream, and bread puddings. Custards and bread puddings are preferred made with evaporated milk. Children drink milk; adults only use it to sweeten their beverages.

Cereal products include rice and rice puddings, sopspaillas, and tortillas, the last made with a flour called masa that is soaked in lime before grinding, which increases its calcium content.

Few fruit varieties are consumed. Mangoes are a favorite as are nopales, a cactus or prickly pear fruit. Chilis are the most commonly used vegetable, with corn, tomatoes, potatoes, and perhaps a few greens accompanying them, often cooked or fried in lard.

Mexican Americans love sweetened beverages. These can be chocolate, coffee, or carbonated drinks. They also love cookies, sweet rolls, donuts, or a little cake called pan de dulce. These are popular after meals, between meals, and before bedtime.

Breakfast is usually tortillas, often served with fried beans, eggs or cereal, and a beverage. Lunch menus used to be similar to those served at dinner and consisted of beans and rice, bread or tortillas, meat or sausage, often as some one-pot stew, perhaps a vegetable or lettuce and tomato, and a beverage. Newer lunch patterns include soup, sandwich, coffee or soft drink, and perhaps a fruit but dinners remain traditional.

Overall, the diet has good sources of Vitamins A and C in the chilis and tomatoes, but now less chilis and tomatoes are being eaten. The consumption of full fat cheeses and evaporated milk that contain calcium, riboflavin, and protein is also on the decline. Tortillas were always made from masa; those made from wheat flour are increasing in popularity and as such are not a good source of calcium.

Greater use of green and yellow vegetables needs to be encouraged as does the use of enriched flour and cereal products, more poultry, fish, and fruits. A reduction in lard use, carbonated beverages, and sweet snacks and an increase in the consumption of milk, preferably that with low fat are recommended.

3.1.2 Puerto Rican Americans

Another large Hispanic group are those from Puerto Rico. In the decade from 1970 to 1980, there was a 40% increase in their population which brought their numbers in the United States to about two million, almost half of them second- or third-generation residents. They and even newer immigrants are changing their food habits, eating lots of pizza, hot dogs, canned spaghetti, and cold cereal although they have few problems obtaining foods needed to maintain traditional dietary patterns. These traditional meals are in use at main family and festival meals and always include a short grain, shiny white rice, washed well before cooking, enhanced with lard and salt during the cooking process, and served with beans.

On a daily basis, Puerto Ricans commonly use rice, beans of all colors and varieties, lard, starchy vegetables, bacalao (dried salted codfish), sofrito (sauce of green peppers, tomatoes, and garlic), and coffee. Breakfast is bread and coffee followed by a light lunch of rice and/or beans or one or more starchy vegetables with or without codfish. There is typically a very late dinner at nine or ten in the evening that includes rice, beans, starchy vegetables, a little chicken or pork, if affordable, and a thick soup often flavored with bacalao.

The lunch pattern is changing; more recently it consists of soup and/or sandwich and coffee or carbonated beverage. The dinner meal, however, remains as it was.

Frequent snacking is common throughout the day and evening, particularly among children. Snack items include some fruit and heavily sweetened fruit juices, crackers, chocolate milk, bread with jam, and others of low nutrient density.

Common starchy items, many are vegetables, in the Puerto Rican diet include green bananas, green or yellow plaintains, breadfruits, yams or sweet potatoes, and sometimes cassava. These, along with the ever-present rice and beans, and the extensive use of lard, olive oil, sugar, canned fruits, and canned soups make up much of their diet. Except for bacalao, fish use is limited as is the use of meats and poultry. When they are served, the portions are small.

There is very limited use of green leafy vegetables. Milk is little used except by very young children. As indicated in the discussion of Mexican Americans above, adults like it only in their strong coffee or in cocoa where several ounces may be added along with a large helping of sugar. They also use it in very sweet pudding type desserts.

Some practices of the "hot-cold" theory show Puerto Rican acceptance of current thinking mixed with older traditional practices. One example is that milk is now considered an important part of a child's diet and ifa child has a cold, considered a hot illness, then milk, a food classified as cold by the hot-cold therapeutic system, is withheld from the child. However, milk is not given to the child with a fever, though fever is considered a hot disease. Other examples can be found in the References. Needless to say, understanding traditional beliefs and newly accepted thinking is complex.

When both parents work, family members frequently eat breakfast separately and hurriedly. Lunch is necessarily consumed at work or at school. Dinner is still served at a late hour, with rice and beans the core of the meal.

Studies have shown that with changes in dietary patterns have come increased rates of high blood pressure, diabetes, ulcers, and other gastro-intestinal disorders. Studies have also shown that Puerto Rican and other Hispanic Americans are marginally deficient in many major nutrients including calcium, vitamin A, riboflavin, and folic acid, they are not deficient in calories. When body weight assessment and skin-fold measures are taken, values are high, indicating obesity.

Nutritional objectives should involve maintenance of ideal body weight, encouragement of use of low-fat dairy products, increased consumption of unsugared fruit juices, and greater variety in preparation and choice of vegetables. Sugar and other simple carbohydrates and the excessive use of fats in cooking should be discouraged.

3.1.3 Cuban Americans

Cuban preferences and food patterns are similar to those groups from the West Indies where Spanish influences predominate. Rice and beans are staples, starchy roots and tubers are popular, and meat is used only when the income allows it. Many fruits and vegetables are consumed as are sweetened beverages and desserts. Cuban Americans like to snack, and do so frequently. Milk is served to children, some even consume too much of it. Adults only use it in coffee, ice cream, other desserts, and in a limited number of cheese products.

3.1.4 Overall

The main foods of Hispanic American populations include high use of starchy vegetables and legumes. Milk use is usually limited, obesity a problem, low nutriture a concern in some populations, and use of fruits and vegetables less than recommended. For nutrient composition of foods specific to these ethnic groups consult the Tables of Food Composition.

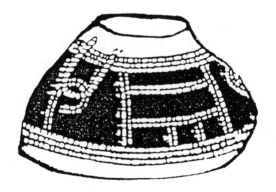

3.2 References

Abraiva, C., A.M. Lawrence, B.A. Nemchausky, S. Sontag, and A.M. Gordon. "Letters to the editor on field study on health and nutrition of Cuban refugees." AMER. J. CLIN. NUTR. 36 (1983): 1255-1259.

Detailed letter to the editor takes issue with previous observations on health and nutrition of Cuban refugees. The authors, responding to a study reported in Volume 35, pages 582-590, defend conclusions and methodology shedding additional light on nutrition and health of the Cuban population.

Acosta, A., M. Amar, S.C. Cornbluth-Szarfarc, E. Dillman, M. Fosil, R.G. Biachi, G. Grebe, E. Hertrampf, S. Kremenchuzky, M. Layrisse, C. Martinez-Torres, C. Moron, F. Pizarro, C. Reynafarje, A. Stekel, D. Villavicencio, and H. Zuniga. "Iron absorption from typical Latin American diets." AMER. J. CLIN. NUTR. 39 (1984): 857-871.

Extrinsic label method is used to determine iron absorption in typical diets consumed in Argentina, Brazil, Chile, Mexico, Peru, and Venezuela. It reveals sevenfold differences that are attributed to varied absorption enhancers such as meat or inhibitors such as tea, wheat, or maize.

Acosta, P.B. "Mexican American low-income groups." PRACTICES OF LOW-INCOME FAMILIES IN FEEDING INFANTS AND SMALL CHILDREN. Rockville, MD: USDHEW Public Health Service, 1972, pp. 75-87.

Reviews history of immigrants to California and their attitudes toward food and food practices. Tables show results of various studies, including those on hot and cold foods, foods used during pregnancy, and foods in infants' and childrens' diets thought by Mexican Americans to be harmful.

Acosta, P.B., R.G. Aranda, J.S. Lewis, and M. Read. "Nutritional status of Mexican American preschool children in a border town." AMER. J. CLIN. NUTR. 27 (1974): 1359-1368.

In the group of one-third of the 171 children have heights one or more standard deviations below the mean of Iowa Growth Standards and one-fourth of the weights are below the 16th percentile. Eleven percent do not meet two-thirds RDA for calcium, 44% do not for iron, 13% do not for thiamin, none for riboflavin, 23% do not for preformed niacin, 7% do not for vitamin A, and 29% do not meet two-thirds RDA for ascorbic acid. Some 90% of the children need dental care and a high percentage have not been immunized. The rate of childhood diseases is higher than that generally found in the United States.

Adad, V., J. Ramos, and E. Boyce. "A model for delivery of mental health services to Spanish-speaking minorities." AMER. J. ORTHOPSYCHIAT. 44 (1974): 548-595.

Cultural and linguistic characteristics are shown to be responsive to the population needs. Discusses use of bilingual staff, walk-in clinic, educational and preventative programs, collaboration with faith healers, and cooperation of local political and religious leaders. Emphasis is on the Puerto Rican population.

Aday, L.A., G.Y. Chiu, and R. Anderson. "Methodological issues in health care surveys of the Spanish heritage population." AMER. J. PUBLIC HEALTH 70 (1980): 367-374.

Paper examines national survey data on access to medical care of persons of Spanish heritage. Findings indicate heterogeneity of the groups and the tendency of these populations to say yes to health care attitude questions.

Adelman, J.D. "Staff awareness of Hispanic health beliefs that affect patient compliance with cancer treatment." PROG. CLIN. BIOL. RES. 121 (1983): 85-86.

Non-compliance due to culturally derived beliefs, attitudes, and behaviors should be incorporated into training sessions for the health care staff.

Alvarez, R.J., J.A. Koburger, and H. Appledorf. "Nutritional and microbial changes during production of tostones (fried plantains)." J. FD. PROTEC. 44 (1981): 9-12.

Slicing, soaking in brine, frying, drying, flattening, and refrying are the processes used to prepare plantain. Finished product contains 48% carbohydrate, 21.5% fat, 2.5% protein, and 395 calories per 100 grams. Bacillus and penicillium organisms have been isolated in laboratory samples of plantains.

Baca, J.E. "Some health beliefs of the Spanish speaking." AMER. J. NURS. 69 (1969): 2172-2176.

Discusses psychological and physical diseases, their belief in "organ displacement" as a classification of illness, and a few folk treatments.

Bailey, L.B., P.A. Wagner, C.G. Davis, and J.S. Dinning. "Food frequency related to folacin status in adolescents." J. AMER. DIETET. ASSOC. 847 (1984): 801-804.

See under Black American References.

Bailey, L.B., P.A. Wagner, G.J. Christakis, C.G. Davis, H. Appledorf, P.E. Araujo, E. Dorsey, and J.S. Dinning. "Folacin and iron status and hematological findings in Black and Spanish American adolescents from urban low-income households." AMER. J. CLIN. NUTR. 35 (1982): 1023-1032.

See under Black American References.

Berkanovic, E. "The effect of inadequate language translation on Hispanic responses to health surveys." AMER. J. PUBLIC HEALTH 70 (1980): 1273-1276.

Points to need for back-translation or translating a survey into Spanish then having someone else translate it back into English. Studies without it are less reliable. An additional problem is that non-idiomatic Spanish does not affect the meaning of the translation but does appear to affect the seriousness with which the interview situations are perceived.

Bogardus, E.S. THE MEXICAN IN THE UNITED STATES. New York: Arno Press, 1970. (This is reprint of 1934 edition published by University of Southern California Press.)

Provides a view of problems encountered early by this population, and reveals a particularly lucid understanding and view of the life and health problems of migrant labor camps.

Bowering, J. "Infant nutrition in East Harlem." HUMAN ECOL. 6,4 (1976): 16-19.

See under Black American References.

Bowering, J., R.L. Lowenberg, and M.A. Morrison. "Nutritional status of pregnant women in East Harlem." AMER. J. CLIN. NUTR. 33 (1980): 1987-1996.

See under Black American References.

Brittin, H.C., and D.W. Zinn. "Meat-buying practices of Caucasians, Mexican Americans, and Negroes." J. AMER. DIETET. ASSOC. 71 (1977): 623-628.

See under Black American References.

Burma, J.H., editor. MEXICAN AMERICANS IN THE UNITED STATES:
A READER. New York: Harper and Row, 1970.

A multiplicity of points of view about Mexican Americans on topics such as:
general characteristics, education, religion, social and political behavior, accul-
turaton, and concepts of illness; contains recommendations for those working
with this population that tends to seek help from an outside group only after
all else fails.

Campbell, S. "Folk lore and food habits." CAJANUS 8,4 (1972): 223-236.

Presents Jamaican food habits, lists food fads, describes superstitions, and
has commentary. Explains why faddism is part of the culture and mentions
popularity of herb treatments. Ends with two common tonic recipes and several
reasons for some individual beliefs.

Cardenas, J., C.E. Gibbs, and E.A. Young. "Nutritional beliefs and practices
in primigravid Mexican American women." J. AMER. DIETET. ASSOC.
69 (1976): 262-265.

Investigates 131 patients during initial clinic visit. Findings indicate over
half manifest anemia. Calcium and vitamin A intakes are low. Pica is not seen
frequently, obesity is. Women have little information or insight about foods
as sources of nutrients; considerable confusion regarding maternal weight gain,
child's birth weight, and proper diet.

Chase, H.P., K.M. Hambidge, S.E. Barnett, M.J. Houts-Jacobs, K. Lenz,
and J. Gillespie. "Low vitamin A and zinc concentrations in Mexican
American migrant children with growth retardation." AMER. J. CLIN.
NUTR. 33 (1980): 2346-2349.

Nutritional evaluations of 102 preschool children whose height, weight, or
head circumference are below the third percentile show that 35% have low serum
vitamin A concentrations, 29% show low hair zinc, and 37% have low plasma
zinc.

Coe, S. "Aztec cuisine." PETITS PROPOS CUL. 19 (1985): 11-22.

Discusses origins of Mexican cuisine, festivals, and prohibitions. A second
article to follow will discuss foods, a third, cooking equipment, methods, and
recipes.

Cohen, R. "Principles of preventive mental health programs for ethnic minority populations: The acculturation of Puerto Ricans to the United
States." AMER. J. PSYCHIAT. 128 (1972): 1529-1533.

Author discusses methods and techniques that health services can use to harmonize with value orientations. Problems of adaptation, conceptual framework, design, and implementation of programs can improve psychological and social adjustment of immigrant populations. Table compares Puerto Rican and middle-class American values. Other illustrative materials highlight these issues.

Cosper, B.A., D.E. Hayslip, and S.B. Foree. "The effect of nutrition education on dietary habits of fifth-graders." J. SCHOOL HEALTH 47 (1977): 475-477.

After eight nutrition education lessons, post-dietary intakes reveal only slight changes from pre-dietary period. Eighty-three percent of the subjects have diets that meet less than half of the RDA before instruction, 88% after instruction. This may be attributed to incorrect responses or to the fact that dieting was encouraged for the obese.

CURRENT PUBLICATIONS AND AUDIO-VISUALS OF THE CARIBBEAN FOOD AND NUTRITION INSTITUTE. P.O. Box 140, Kingston, Jamaica, 1982.

Catalogue of 40 items for sale includes those on breast feeding, weaning, anemia, obesity, diabetes, food composition, etc. All are annotated.

Currier, R.L. "The hot-cold syndrome and symbolic balance in Mexican and Spanish American folk medicine." ETHNOLOGY 5 (1966): 251-263.

Discusses health beliefs of these populations. Highlights specific illnesses that are hot or cold and shows how Mexicans and/or Spanish Americans believe them to relate to the social environment. These, combined with child-rearing practices and social relationships, indicate how continued beliefs in the hot-cold concept are fostered.

Day, M.L., M. Lenter, and S. Jaquez. "Food acceptance patterns of Spanish speaking New Mexicans." J. NUTR. EDUC. 10 (1978): 121-123.

Forty women interviewed give frequency and reasons for using foods they consume. Health is selected only 4.6% of the time. Sensory, economic, geographic, and preparation reasons, religion, race, and culture are the most frequently mentioned. Milk, margarine, coffee or tea, enriched breads, onion, citrus fruit juices, and eggs are served daily, and ground beef, luncheon meats, and steaks weekly by 50% or more of the respondents.

de Aponte, I.P. "Family food in Puerto Rico." PARENTS MAG. 3 (1962): 75-76 and 130-132.

Short article details shopping and eating practices and includes 11 recipes for foods mentioned.

Delgaldo, M. "Hispanic natural support systems: Implications for mental health services." J. PSYCHOSOC. NURS. MENT. HEALTH SERV. 21,4 (1983): 19-24.

Important cultural values include extended family, folk healers, religious institutions, merchants, and social clubs. Article indicates preference of Hispanics for less formal relationships between helper/helpee, their disdain for elaborate intake procedures, need to be actively involved in solutions, and desire for concrete tasks. Lists all the cultural values that must be operational to meet the needs of this group.

de Slosser, H. "Food among Puerto Rican families." FOCUS ON MARKETS (N.Y.S. Cooperative Extension at Cornell University), April, 1978.

Discusses how food is served and food's role as a medium of friendship. Typical dinner menus include rice and beans as the core; lunch, if eaten at all, includes canned spaghetti, canned soups, or sandwiches.

Dewey, K.G., M.A. Strode, and Y.R. Fitch. "Anthropometry of migrant and nonmigrant Mexican American children and adults in northern California." ECOL. FD. NUTR. 14 (1984): 25-35.

Growth status of children is related to maternal weight, height, and family income. Among adults in this study of 140 families, 55% of the women and 43% of the men exceed 120% of "ideal" weight. Obesity increases with age but is unrelated to length of residence in the United States.

Dewey, K.G., M.A. Strode, and Y.R. Fitch. "Dietary change among migrant and non-migrant Mexican American families in northern California." ECOL. FD. NUTR. 14 (1984): 11-24.

Preschool children of 140 families have average consumption of all food groups except for low consumption of vegetables. Most adults say their diets have improved since moving to the United States. More migrants than nonmigrants have traditional beliefs proscribing certain foods during illness, pregnancy, or lactation.

Dewey, K.G., E.S. Metallinos, M.A. Strode, E.M. All, Y.R. Fitch, M. Holguin, J.A Kraus, and L.J. McNicholas. "Combining nutrition research and nutrition education – Dietary change among Mexican American families." J. NUTR. EDUC. 16 (1984): 5-7.

Interviews of 40 migrant families reveal 28% work six months or less per year. Overall nutritional quality of the children's diets are good, with four servings of red meat and two of chicken per week, and two to three servings of milk, two of fruits, and one of vegetables per day. Breast feeding is practiced less since coming to the United States, fruit and vegetable consumption is higher. Generally, the families do not purchase foods that they are not familiar with or do not recognize.

DIET MANUAL FOR THE CARIBBEAN. Available from: Caribbean Food and Nutrition Institute, P.O. Box 140, Kingston 7, Jamaica.

Manual details foods and nutrition information specific to this population.

Dominguez, V.R. FROM NEIGHBOR TO STRANGER: THE DILEMMA OF CARIBBEAN PEOPLES IN THE UNITED STATES. New Haven: Yale University Antilles Research Program Occasional Papers 5, 1975.

Dimensions of Caribbean migration to the United States concentrate on those from British West Indies, Haiti, Dominican Republic, Cuba, and Puerto Rico. Book is compilation of data collected from Masters and Doctoral theses with relevent bibliography, general materials, social data, and readings on ethnicity, race, and groups.

Dowd, J.J., and V.L. Bengston. "Aging in minority populations, an examination of the double jeopardy hypothesis." J. GERONTOL. 33 (1978): 427-436.

See under Black American References.

Duncan, B., A.N. Smith, and F.W. Briese. "Comparison of growth: Spanish-surnamed with non-Spanish-surnamed children." AMER. J. PUBLIC HEALTH 69 (1979): 903-907.

Boys and girls with Spanish surnames weigh less, are shorter, and have smaller head circumferences than other children living in the same neighborhoods. Those in lower and lower-middle income neighborhoods are more similar in size no matter what the surname.

Duran, L.I., and H.R. Bernard, editors. INTRODUCTION TO CHICANO STUDIES. New York: Macmillan Co., 1977.

Volume discusses ancient and historical roots of culture, customs, beliefs, social structure, and attempts to control their own destiny. Includes chapters on folk medicine and on the intercultural jest.

Duyff, R.L., D. Sanjur, and H.Y. Nelson. "Food behavior and related factors of Puerto Rican American teen-agers." J. NUTR. EDUC. 7 (1975): 99-103.

Questionnaire responses and three-day food intakes of 75 girls in Chicago show vitamin C intake higher than other teen populations, calcium and iron substantial, and vitamin A levels low due to little intake of vegetables. Low nutriture and high calorie snack food consumption is seen in working teens. Diet is related to knowledge and socioeconomic variables.

Fernandez, N.A. "Nutrition in Puerto Rico." CANCER RES. 35 (1975): 3272-3291.

Gives general information about the island, describes past nutrition research, and lists current foods consumed. Reviews recent research findings in urban and rural areas, and comments on nutrition and cancer in Puerto Rico.

Fernandez, N.A., J.C. Burgos, C.F. Asenjo, and I. Rosa. "Nutritional status of the Puerto Rican population: Master sample survey." AMER. J. CLIN. NUTR. 24 (1971): 952-965.

Surveys 877 families in Puerto Rico and details diet, clinical, and biochemical tests. Higher economic standards do not necessarily improve nutritional value of the diet. Food between meals is consumed by 76.5%, codfish a staple in the diet of about the same percent, and starchy vegetables the bulk of the diet for all. Fruit consumption is low, rice the favorite grain, and lard the preferred fat. Greater levels of nutrient deficiency appear in people with higher incomes and are accompanied by a high prevalence of excess weight.

FOOD CONSUMPTION AND DIETARY LEVELS OF HOUSEHOLDS IN PUERTO RICO, SUMMER AND FALL 1977, Preliminary Report # 9. Hyattsville, MD: United States Department of Agriculture, 1982.

Fifty-six percent of the 2,976 households do major food purchasing less than once a week, 46% participate in the food stamp program and 33% of their food dollar is spent on meat, poultry, and fish. On average, the diets are sufficient to provide food energy; 11 other nutrients evaluated. RDA's for vitamin A and calcium are somewhat low.

FOOD IS GOOD. Yakima, WA: Yakima Home Economics Association, 1973.

Six booklets in Spanish or English are available in a nutrition series for young children. There is also a videotape available with the same title. They contain illustrations and questions and activities revolving around a few basic concepts.

Garcia-Palmieri, M.R., M. Sorlie, J. Tillotson, R. Costas, E. Cordero, and M. Rodriguez. "Relationship of dietary intake to subsequent coronary heart incidence: The Puerto Rico heart health program." AMER. J. CLIN. NUTR. 33 (1980): 1818-1827.

Study of 8,218 urban and rural men ages 45 to 64 show urban diets significantly higher in total fat and lower in calorie and carbohydrate intake. Urban men who develop myocardial infarction have lower calorie and carbohydrate intakes than do the rural men. Multivariate analysis demonstrates an independent inverse relation of carbohydrate intake from legumes to coronary heart disease incidence. Dietary sucrose shows no relationship.

Gardner, L.I., Jr., M.P. Stern, S.M. Haffner, S.P. Gaskill, H.P. Hazuda, H.J. Relethford, and C.F. Eifler. "Prevalence of diabetes in Mexican Americans: Relationship to percent of gene pool derived from native American sources." DIABETES 33 (1984): 86-95.

The association of genetic admixture with non-insulin-dependent diabetes mellitus suggests that much of the epidemic of this form of diabetes is confined to that part of the population with substantial native American heritage.

Garn, S.M., and M. LaVelle. "Reproductive histories of low weight girls and women." AMER. J. CLIN. NUTR. 37 (1983): 862-866.

Four different studies of nearly 80,000 women show low body weight is especially common in Puerto Rican and Mexican American girls who mature early.

Giachello, A.L., R. Bell, L.A. Aday, and R.M. Anderson. "Uses of the 1980 census for Hispanic health services research." AMER. J. PUBLIC HEALTH 73 (1983): 266-274.

Describes how census data assists in estimating health care needs. Indicates that while far from adequate or ideal, this data is often the best available source and should be used. Several methods are suggested.

Gordon, A.M. "Nutritional status of Cuban refugees: A field study on the health and nutriture of refugees processed at Opa Locka, Florida." AMER. J. CLIN. NUTR. 35 (1982): 582-590.

Field study evaluates 138 newly arrived refugees and reveals that 25% of children suffer malnutrition, 17% of the women are obese, and 15% of women and 12% of children have anemia. Foods most frequently consumed exclude fruits and vegetables and include bread, rice, eggs, and garbanzo beans (chick peas).

GUIDELINES TO FOOD AND DIETARY SERVICES IN THE CONTEM-
PORARY CARIBBEAN, Report of CFNI Technical Group Meeting.
Kingston, Jamaica: Caribbean Food and Nutrition Institute, 1975.

Gives organization, training, menu planning, purchasing, storage, and other organizational features of dietary departments. Provides list of individuals and addresses for locating food and nutrition information.

Gurney, J.M. "Nutritional considerations concerning the staple foods of the English-speaking Caribbean." ECOL. FOOD NUTR. 4 (1975): 171-175.

Staple foods include wheat, rice, maize, starchy fruits, some roots and tubers, and sugar. They are listed in terms of energy and protein value of the Caribbean diet.

Harwood, A. "The hot-cold theory of disease." J. AMER. MED. ASSOC. 216 (1971): 1153-1158.

Overview of illnesses, medicines, and foods. Includes some historical background, patient behaviors, use of medications, and means of communication with patients holding hot-cold beliefs. Examples highlight patient dilemmas when fruit juices are recommended for a cold and the patient's culture suggests hot ginger tea.

Hayes-Bautista, D.E. "Identifying Hispanic populations: The influence of research methodology upon public policy." AMER. J. PUBLIC HEALTH 70 (1980): 353-356.

Editorial suggests research using Hispanic surnames is not reliable to study populations. The birthplace of their parents can be equally faulty. Author offers no solution but details need to clarify terminology beyond those in current vogue, i.e., Hispanic or Spanish surname.

Hope, M. "Taboos about breast feeding." CAJUNUS 8 (1975): 190-193.

Lists some superstitions surrounding breast milk. Prohibitions of milk include: if given to babies at night it sours their stomachs, breast milk from a quarrelling mother is unsuitable for consumption, and milk from a mother who has been sweating will make the baby sick. Also discusses taboos of foods other than breast milk.

Hunt, I.F., N.J. Murphy, A.E. Cleaver, N. Laine, and V.A. Clark. "Protective foods as a tool for dietary assessment in the evaluation of public health programs for pregnant Hispanics." ECOL. FD. NUTR. 12 (1983): 235-245.

Protective Foods Recall, a new tool, includes dietary demerit scoring system. It was developed with recall questionnaire using basic food groupings and additional categories. Discusses the methodology for administration and illustrates with 30 pregnant Hispanic women whose scores show the instrument can be compared to 24 hour dietary recall.

Hunt, I.F., M. Jacob, N.J. Ostergard, G. Masri, V.A. Clark, and A.H. Coulson. "Effect of nutrition education on the nutritional status of low-income pregnant women of Mexican descent." AMER. J. CLIN. NUTR. 29 (1976): 675-684.

A sample of 344 pregnant women reveals benefits of nutrition education. Treatment group shows increase in mean intake of protein, ascorbic acid, niacin, riboflavin, and thiamin, and decrease in incidence of multiple low nutrient intakes. Except for improvement in mean serum folate levels, biochemical indices for the treatment group do not improve.

Hunt, I.F., N.J. Ostergard, L.P. Carroll, B. Hsieh, R. Brown, and V. Gladney. "Iron, thiamin, riboflavin, and niacin content of corn tortillas made in Los Angeles, California." ECOL. FD. NUTR. 7 (1978): 37-39.

Corn tortillas are common food in the diet of people of Mexican descent. Analyzed on a weight basis they have less iron, thiamin, riboflavin, and niacin than enriched white bread. The mean intake of iron, thiamin, and riboflavin of this population is below two-thirds of the RDA and addition of these nutrients is recommended.

Hunt, I.F., N.J. Murphy, A.E. Cleaver, B. Faraji, M.E. Swendseid, A.H. Coulson, V.A. Clark, B.L. Browdy, M.T. Cabalum, and J.C. Smith, Jr. "Zinc supplementation during pregnancy: Effects on selected blood constituents and on progress and outcome of pregnancy in low-income women of Mexican descent." AMER. J. CLIN. NUTR. 40 (1984): 508-521.

Double-blind study of 213 women reveals that with or without zinc supplementation, women with low serum zinc levels have higher mean ribonuclease and lower alpha-amino-levulinic acid dehydratase activity than women with acceptable zinc levels. The incidence of pregnancy induced hypertension is higher in the control group than in the zinc-supplemented group. The expected increase in serum copper levels is greater in women with pregnancy-induced hypertension than in normotensives.

Hunt, I.F., N.J. Murphy, A.E. Cleaver, B. Faraji, M.E. Swendseid, A.H. Coulson, V.A. Clark, N. Laine, C.A. Davis, and J.C. Smith, Jr. "Zinc supplementation during pregnancy: Zinc concentration from serum and hair from low-income women of Mexican descent." AMER. J. CLIN. NUTR. 37 (1983): 572-582.

Initial mean dietary zinc intake of 213 pregnant women is 50% of the RDA. Zinc supplementation does not alter mean zinc levels initially but it does significantly reduce the number of low serum zinc values toward the end of pregnancy

Jacob, M., I.F. Hunt, O. Dirige, and M.E. Swendseid. "Biochemical assessment of the nutritional status of low-income pregnant women of Mexican descent." AMER. J. CLIN. NUTR. 29,6 (1976): 650-656.

Folacin is the most prevalent vitamin deficiency in a group of 300 pregnant women studied; 69% have low or deficient serum levels. In addition, 22% are low in thiamin, 29% in riboflavin, and 9% in pyridoxine. Fewer deficiencies are found in those women taking vitamin and mineral supplements.

King, L.M. "The Spanish speaking American." ETHNIC AMERICAN MINORITIES. Edited and compiled by H.A. Johnson. New York: R.R. Bowker Co., 1976, pp. 189-240.

Includes first a profile of income and age statistics, then details Mexican Americans, Puerto Ricans, and Cubans and finally gives an overview of their cultural needs, styles of reasoning, relationships, family structure, religion, and educational needs. Describes 88 films, 49 filmstrip or filmstrip series, 24 slide or transparency sets, 39 audio or video recordings or cassettes and 11 sets of graphic materials. There is a directory of the producers and distributors.

Knapp, J.A., S.M. Haffner, E.A. Young, H.P. Haduza, L. Gardner, and M.P. Stern. "Dietary intakes of essential nutrients among Mexican Americans and Anglo-Americans: The San Antonio heart study." AMER. J. CLIN. NUTR. 42 (1985): 307-316.

One day recalls of 2,134 residents in three different socioeconomic areas show mean intakes of calcium and vitamins A and C significantly lower among the Mexican Americans and the intake of vitamin C most affected by socioeconomic status. Females of both groups consume less than the RDA for calcium and iron.

Landman, J., and J.S.E. Hall. "The dietary habits and knowledge of folklore of pregnant Jamaican women." ECOL. FD. NUTR. 12 (1983): 203-210.

Results of study of 125 pregnant Jamaican women reflect persistence of traditional folklore. Pregnant women indicate increase in preference for fluids, cravings for salty foods and ice. Pica reports are rare. Relationship to lower socioeconomic status is significant.

Larson, L.B., J.M. Dodds, D.M. Massoth, and H.P. Chase. "Nutritional status of Mexican American migrant families." J. AMER. DIETET. ASSOC. 64 (1974): 29-35.

Vitamin A deficiency is widespread problem in a three year study of 149 families. Nutrients except for Vitamin D, are generally adequate to high. Consumption of foods from the fruit and vegetable, and milk groups is low, iron slightly low, and protein twice the recommended allowance.

Leung, W.T.W. FOOD COMPOSITION TABLE FOR USE IN LATIN AMERICA. Bethesda, MD: Interdepartmental Committee on Nutrition for National Defense, 1961.

See listing under Tables of Food Composition.

Levitt, C., J. Godes, M. Eberhardt, R. Ing, and J.M. Simpson. "Sources of lead poisoning." J. AMER. MED. SOC. 252 (1984): 3127-3128.

Letter reveals that azarcon, a bright orange powder used by Mexican and other Hispanic parents to treat chronic indigestion or "empacho" contains 86 to 93.5% lead tetroxide. Other powders given to other ethnic groups also show high lead content.

Lieberman, L.S. "Medico-nutritional practices among Puerto Ricans in a small urban northeastern community in the United States." SOC. SCI. MED. 138 (1979): 191-198.

Discusses the changes in the Puerto Rican folk medico-nutritional system. Current beliefs, including the hot-cold paradigm, eating patterns, and conflicts in nutrition and health care behaviors show a community that is rapidly acculturating through efforts of cooperative integration of folk and scientific mediconutritional systems.

Linn, M.W., K.I. Hunter, and B.S. Linn. "Self-assessed health,impairment, and disability in Anglo, Black, and Cuban elderly." MED. CARE 18,3 (1980): 7 unnumbered pages.

Comparison of 174 elderly outpatients show differences among cultures. Blacks rate themselves most disabled, Cubans least disabled. Self-assesed health reveals a different pattern with Cubans reporting the poorest levels of health and Anglos, or non-Hispanic whites, the best. The five most frequent medical diagnoses (arthritis, high blood pressure, heart condition, nervous condition, and cataracts) show no statistical differences and are somewhat similar for the three groups of elderly. The patient's estimates of health appears to be an important factor in overall health status.

Marchione, T.J. "A history of breast feeding practices in the English speaking Caribbean." FD. HEALTH BULL. 2 (1980): 9-18.

Mixed feeding of carbohydrate gruels is used by the third or fourth month following birth and these gruels follow bush tea use which begins in the first month. Too early weaning and poor and unsanitary diets are common problems.

Marrs, D.C. "Milk drinkiing by the elderly of three races." J. AMER. DIETET. ASSOC. 72 (1978): 495-498.

See under Black American References.

May, J.M., and D.L. McMellan. THE ECOLOGY OF MALNUTRITION IN THE CARIBBEAN. New York: Hafner Press, 1973.

Volume 12 in the series includes the Bahamas, Cuba, Jamaica, Haiti, Dominican Republic, Puerto Rico, Lesser Antilles, Trinidad, and Tobago and investigates background, food resources, diets, nutritional disease patterns, and related issues. Traditional diets in most of these countries include imported cod, local beans, rice and a rich variety of fruits indicating influence of countries that dominated politically at one time or another; some of the areas having changed foreign domination as many as 14 times.

May, J.M., and D.L. McLellan. THE ECOLOGY OF MALNUTRITION IN WESTERN SOUTH AMERICA. New York: Hafner Press, 1974.

This, volume 14 in the Studies in Medical Geography series, investigates background, food resources, diets, nutritional disease patterns, and related issues of Colombia, Ecuador, Peru, Bolivia, and Chile. Their populations are primarily mestizo and pure-blooded Indians. Except in Chile, food is not always in adequate supply. Chapters on diets and nutritional disease patterns are rich in research in this study sponsored by United States Army.

McKigney, J.I., and R. Cook, editors. PROTEIN FOODS FOR THE CARIBBEAN. Kingston, Jamaica: The Caribbean Food and Nutrition Institute, 1968.

Proceedings of a conference held at Georgetown, Guyana. Eight sessions included background on food and nutrition of the region, availability of protein resources, protein foods, and development and testing of infant weaning foods.

Millard, A.V., and M.A. Graham. "Principles that guide weaning in rural Mexico." ECOL. FD. NUTR. 16 (1985): 171-188.

Decisions in weaning by Mexican women are based on maternal and child health, not the chronological age of the infant. Reasons include: the concern that if child has teeth, the combination of the mother's milk and other food will sicken the child, another pregnancy, presence of strong emotional states such as severe fright, profound anger, or grief, and the belief that a child who is too old who continues to breast feed will grow up to be boorish and ill-mannered.

Padilia, E. UP FROM PUERTO RICO. New York: Columbia University Press, 1958.

Provides detailed description of the ways of life and the changing culture of Puerto Ricans in a New York City slum in terms of what happens to the uprooted family, the children, the health, and the traditions and values. The chapter on health and life stress includes old world and new life views on disease and restoration of health, including hot-cold theories, and recommended cures. Some reference is made to special foods for recovery, diets for health, and foods that "fall well" in the stomach.

Parker, S.L., and J. Bowering. "Folacin in diets of Puerto Rican and Black women in relation to food practices." J. NUTR. EDUC. 8 (1976): 73-76.

See under Black American References.

Powell-Griner, E., and D. Streck. "A closer examination of neonatal mortality rates among the Texas Spanish surname population." AMER. J. PUBLIC HEALTH 72 (1982): 993-999.

During five of the last ten years, neonatal mortality rates for those with Spanish surnames are lower than those for Anglos. Various reasons are discrepanicies in coding of race, in underreporting, and in large number of Mexican residents reported as Texas residents.

RECOMMENDED DIETARY ALLOWANCES FOR THE CARIBBEAN. Kingston, Jamaica: Caribbean Food and Nutrition Institute, 1979.

Summarizes existing FAO/WHO recommendations and comments on historical aspects of deficiency diseases, their clinical description, and the dietary sources of individual nutrients.

Roberts, R.E., and E.S. Lee. "The health of Mexican Americans: Evidence from the human population laboratory studies." AMER. J. PUBLIC HEALTH 70 (1980): 375-384.

Data for 3,776 Mexican Americans are compared to Blacks and Anglos. Blacks report more chronic conditions, more disability, and more symptoms while Chicanos report fewer health problems. The two most powerful predictors of health status are age/sex and perceived health; ethnicity is not a good predictor.

Roberts, R.E., and E.S. Lee. "Medical care use by Mexican Americans." MED. CARE 18,3 (1980): 16 unnumbered pages.

Data from sample surveys of 3,776 living in California compares Mexican Americans to Anglos and Blacks in terms of medical visits, dental, and eye examinations. Very little ethnic difference exists regarding source of medical care or health insurance coverage though fewer Chicanos have such coverage. In terms of visits to physicians, there is little difference between Anglos and Chicanos, Blacks visit physicians most, and more Chicanos than either of the other groups have never had a physical examination. Mexican Americans report the lowest rate of dental examinations and never having had an eye examination.

Ross Laboratories. NUTRITION MATERIALS. Columbus, OH: Ross Educational Services, 1982.

Many materials for breast, bottle feeding, and related nutrition topics available in Spanish and English.

Ruiz, P. "Culture and mental health: A Hispanic perspective." J. CONTEMP. PSYCHOTHERAPY 9,1 (1977): 24-27.

Because folk healing practices include need under stress, a central hospital sets out to learn and teach folk healers symptoms which should be investigated by trained professionals. Once barriers are lowered, they learn from each other in roles of student and teacher enabling coordination of both systems. Development of inservice training sessions expand this knowledge.

Salmon, M.B. LA ALEGRIA DE LA ALIMENTACION A PECHO (THE JOY OF BREASTFEEDING). Demarest, NJ: Techkits, 1984.

Handbook, written in Spanish for parents and health professionals, has pictures and lists of culturally accepted nutritious foods.

Salmon, M.B. DIABETIC DIET EXCHANGE LISTS FOR LOW SODIUM DIETS. Demarest, NJ: Techkits, 1980.

Booklet includes sample menu plan and list of acceptable foods and those to avoid in each of the exchange lists. Also available are DIABETIC EXCHANGE LISTS and DIETA DIABETICA PARA BUENA SALUD, both similar to the above.

Sandoval, M. "Santeria: Afrocuban concepts of disease and its treatment in Miami." J. OPER. PSYCHIATRY 8,2 (1977): 52-63.

Santeria, an Afro-Cuban religious system, is described in terms of beliefs of disease cause, the power of plants, herbs, and weeds, and the success of adjustment in an industrial and technical society. Illustrations heighten explanations of supernatural causes, important gods, and the therapeutic value of potions made from vegetation that grows only in the wild. A list of uses for some of them is given with Afro-Cuban, Spanish, English, and Latin names.

Schulman, S., and A.M. Smith. "The concept of health among Spanish speaking villagers of New Mexico and Colorado." J. HEALTH HUMAN BEHAV. 4 (1963): 226-234.

The identification of healthy is based on folk medical system of isolated villagers. Criteria for health are high level of physical activity, a well-fleshed body, and an absence of pain.

Selby, M.L., E.S. Lee, D.M. Tuttle, and H.D. Loe, Jr. "Validity of Spanish surname infant mortality rate as a health status indicator for the Mexican American population." AMER. J. PUB. HEALTH 74 (1984): 998-1002.

Spanish surname infant mortality rate may be low and does not appear to be a valid indicator of Mexican American health status. Findings suggest infant death data are compatible with migration and underregistration of deaths.

Shaloub, J., and C. Murray. CLINICAL SPANISH FOR DIETITIANS. Fullerton, CA.: Plycon Press, 1977.

Extensive alphabetical list includes food items, phrases commonly used to greet patients, and sentences needed to discuss health and food history. The sentences are organized by diet type or nutrient source. A short dictionary for quick reference is included. All are given in English to Spanish and Spanish to English.

Simmons, W.K., and M.J. Gurney. "Nutritional anemia in the English-speaking Caribbean and Suriname." AMER. J. CLIN. NUTR. 34 (1981): 327-337.

Anemia is common in areas studied and mostly affects preschool children, pregnant and lacting women. Common causes are inadequate intake and a deficiency of folate, less common is anemia associated with parasitic infestation.

Simoni, J.J., L.A. Vargas, and L. Casillas. "Merolicos and health education." BULL. PAN AMER. HEALTH ORG. 17,1 (1983): 4-18.

Five merolicos or medicine men were given some nutrition education on the care of infants and children. Two months later interviews with girls ages 11 to 19 who had seen these men indicate that most had remembered the instruction and put it into practice. This is a compelling argument for support of medicine men in some public health programs.

SPANISH LANGUAGE MATERIALS FOR PEOPLE WITH DIABETES. NIH Publication No. 81-2180. Bethesda, MD: National Diabetes Clearing House, 1981.

Selected annotations of available materials. Lists of food by type and portion are given in Spanish as are suggested menus with calorie counts.

Stephenson, S. "Ole! The Mexican craze catches fire." FD. MGT. 14 (1979): 52+.

Discusses popularity of Mexican food in schools and colleges, merchandising ideas, and quantity recipies.

Stern, M.P., J.A. Pugh, S.P. Gaskill, and H.P. Hazuda. "Knowledge, attitudes, and behavior related to obesity and dieting in Mexican Americans and Anglos: The San Antonio heart study." AMER. J. EPIDEM. 115 (1982): 917-927.

Study was carried out in two middle and upper income areas and found that Mexican Americans were leaner than their lower income counterparts but more overweight than the Anglos. Mexican Americans of both sexes agree with the statement that Americans are too concerned about weight loss.

Stern, M.P., W.L. Haskell, P.D.S. Wood, K.E. Osann, A.B. King, and J.W. Farquhar. "Affluence and cardiovascular risk factors in Mexican Americans and other Whites in three northern California communities." J. CHRON. DIS. 28 (1975): 623-636.

Survey of 1,666 randomly selected men and women reveals that 17.9% of the Mexican Americans have plasma cholesterol levels and blood pressure similar to that of Whites. The latter have greater adiposity and higher plasma triglyceride levels though fewer are heavy smokers and more consume alcohol. Adiposity is correlated with blood pressure and plasma triglycerides in both ethnic groups.

Torres, R.M. "Dietary patterns of the Puerto Rican people." AMER. J. CLIN. NUTR. 7 (1959): 349-355.

Description of typical diet includes reasons for consumption or avoidance of certain foods. Details common starchy food items such as plaintains and cassava, and includes a table of nutritional value for 14 of them. Includes typical meal plan, values for the common starchy foods on diabetic exchange lists, diet modifications, holiday foods, and a glossary.

United States Department of Education. BIBLIOGRAPHY. Kansas City, MO: Region VII Refugees Materials Center, 1983.

Materials available from the center include hundreds of items geared to many ethnic groups. One section lists those for Spanish-speaking refugees and includes teaching materials, language items, first aid, and general items needed for adjusting to a new location.

Valverde, V., I. Nieves, N. Sloan, B. Pillet, F. Trowbridge, T. Farrell, I. Beghin, and R.E. Klein. "Lifestyles and nutritional status of children from different ecological areas of El Salvador." ECOL. FD. NUTR. 9 (1980): 167-177.

Data includes characteristics of the population and its lifestyles, diets of children from birth to five years, and height and weight information. Practices include: use of cinnamon flavored water fed to babies three days old, breast feeding of children usually to about 12 months, and orange juice and oat gruel placed in the bottle for babies at one month of age.

Varela, G., O. Moreiras-Varela, and A. Requejo. "Vitamin status of the Spanish population." ACTA. VITAMIN. ENZYMOL. 4,1-2 (1982): 123-133.

Vitamin consumption in several Spanish population groups is satisfactory except for vitamin A and riboflavin. People with low incomes or on reducing diets are among those who may be at risk. Comparisons are made with other countries and table is included about intake recomendations for 10 countries.

Vilhjalmsdottir, L., A.G. Ferris, V.A. Beal, and P.L. Pellett. "Short stature and overweight in infants of western Massachusetts." ECOL. FD. NUTR. 8 (1979): 127-135.

See under Black American References.

Weaver, J.L "Mexican American health care behavior: A critical review of the literature." SOC. SCI. QUARTERLY 54 (1973): 85-102.

Stresses the importance of anthropological and sociological research findings and the means of avoiding common methodological shortcomings in research and treatment of this population group. Forty Mexican American health care studies are reviewed. Discussion details common and less common practices.

Wilson, C.S. "Nutrition education and the Spanish-speaking American: An annotated bibliography (1961-1972)." J. NUTR. EDUC. 5, Supplement 1 (1973): 161-179.

Food and nutrition, consumer problems, and other health related topics are annotated. There are sections on printed materials, audiovisuals, and materials about Spanish-speaking people in the Americas. Lists hundreds of English and Spanish materials, all with annotations in English.

Woteki, C.E., E. Weser, and E.A. Young. "Lactose malabsorption in Mexican American adults." AMER. J. CLIN. NUTR. 30 (1977): 470-475.

Lactose malabsorption is found in 53% of the Mexican Americans and 15% of the Anglo-Americans in a group of 419 adults ages 18 to 94. Milk and dairy product consumption is the same in both ethnic groups, as is general intake of protein, calories, riboflavin, vitamin A, and calcium. Nearly 60% of the Mexican American and 24% of the Anglo-American malabsorbers experience recognizable symptoms after milk consumption.

Yetley, E.A., M.J. Yetley, and B. Aguirre. "Family role structure and food related roles in Mexican American families." J. NUTR. EDUC. 13, Supplement 1 (1981): 96-101.

Sex stereotypes are not well supported in this study as men are involved in food purchase decisions and women in money decisions. Rethinking is necessary when planning education programs for this ethnic group.

Yokai, F. "Dietary pattern of Spanish speaking people living in the Boston area." J. AMER. DIETET. ASSOC. 71 (1977): 273-275.

Using Puerto Rican, Cuban, Mexican and other common Hispanic food, nutrition counseling suggestions include decreasing carbonated beverage and beer intake, not cooking vegetables in animal fat, and increasing calcium consumption.

Zavaleta, A.N., and R.M. Malina. "Growth, fatness, and leanness in Mexican American children." AMER. J. CLIN. NUTR. 33 (1980): 2008-2020.

Mexican American children compare favorably with others in the Health Examination Survey, their diet is adequate in calories but less satisfactory in protein. About five to seven percent are obese.

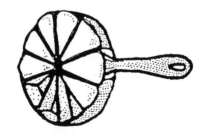

3.3 Resources for Recipes

Aaron, J. THE ART OF MEXICAN COOKING. Garden City, NY: Doubleday & Co., Inc., 1965.

Includes influences of the cuisine and a glossary of ingredients. Additional information precedes each main food ingredient chapter. All recipes are titled with local name and English translation, and all were gathered in Mexico. A short chapter on fiesta foods concludes the book.

Bensusan, S. LATIN AMERICAN COOKING. New York: Galahad Books 1973.

Generalized background information precede recipes culled from all of Central and South America; country of origin listed only in the index. Most recipes have color photograph of the completed dish.

de Andrade, M. BRAZILIAN COOKERY, TRADITIONAL AND MODERN. Rutland, VT: Charles E. Tuttle Co., 1965.

Recipes show native Indian, Portuguese, and Negro slave influences. There is one chapter on Afro-Brazilian cookery, the rest are given by food category with many of the recipes common to other countries of Central and South America.

de Leon, J.V. MEXICAN COOK BOOK. Mexico City, Mexico: Culinary Arts Institute, 1956.

Recipes from every region of Mexico are adapted for use in United States and are written in Spanish and English. First part of the book explains vocabulary, utensils, and other background materials. Recipes follow and are divided by main ingredient with one section giving recipes by regions with in Mexico.

Grey, W. CARIBBEAN COOKING. London: Collins Publications, 1965.

Using advice of dietitians and home economists in the Caribbean, book begins with a short introductory giving nutrient content of common local fruits and vegetables. Recipes are divided by main food ingredients with last chapters on sweets in many forms, traditional West Indian dishes, cooking for invalids, leftovers, table service, and reference charts.

Kaufman, W.I., editor. RECIPES FROM THE CARIBBEAN AND LATIN AMERICA. New York: Dell Publishing Co., 1964.

Paperback has 300 specialities from 27 countries, each listing country of origin. Recipes, adapted for American ingredients and kitchens, are grouped in chapters by main ingredient. Index is alphabetical and by country.

Kennedy, D. THE CUISINES OF MEXICO. New York: Harper & Row, 1972.

Thorough details of Mexican kitchen, ingredients, chilis, and cooking methods begin the book. This is followed by recipes, sources for ingredients, pronunciation guide, and bibliography.

Kennedy, D. THE TORTILLA BOOK. New York: Harper & Row, 1975.

Large paperback devotes considerable space to background material. Recipes are given for corn not wheat tortillas of Mexico and include those for every course in a meal.

Kirshman, I., editor. LATIN AMERICAN COOKING. New York: Galahad Books, 1973.

Short introduction includes background information. This is followed by recipes, some with colored photographs, divided by food category and not indicating country of origin. This is one of 12 titles in the 'ROUND THE WORLD COOKING LIBRARY series.

Leonard, J.N. LATIN AMERICAN COOKING. New York: Time-Life Books, 1970.

Central and South American cookery details roots and current practices. Chapters are divided according to heritages. Recipes appear in this and in the companion RECIPES: LATIN AMERICAN COOKING volume, neither gives country of origin.

Maze, C.M. MEXICAN MICROWAVE COOKERY. Las Cruces, NM: Bilingue Publications, 1984.

Intention is to transfer time-consuming Mexican recipes to preparation in the microwave oven. Recipes are by food category and appear after short sections on oven use, substitutions, and hints about Mexican cookery.

Mulvey, R.W., and L.M. Alvarez. GOOD FOOD FROM MEXICO. New York: Collier Books, 1968.

Short background precedes 350 recipes for every occasion – barbecue to feast – given in food category chapters. Glossary of unusual ingredients appears at the end.

Slater, M. CARIBBEAN COOKING FOR PLEASURE. London: Hamlyn, 1970.

Short introduction and glossary precede recipes in food category chapters. No countries of origin are listed.

Stone, S., and M. Stone. CLASSIC MEXICAN COOKING. New York: A Wallaby Book, 1985.

Short introduction followed by recipes in chapters by food category in this paperback.

Valdejuli, C.A. PUERTO RICAN COOKERY. Santurce, PR: By the author, 1977.

Many editions of this volume, 34 at last count, make it the "Joy of Cooking" of Puerto Rico. Recipes are given by food category; a glossary explains unusual items.

Vazquez-Prego, A. HOW ARGENTINA COOKS. Buenos Aires, Argentina: El Ateneo, 1979.

Bilingual volume of recipes with chapters by food category includes cultural information where applicable. Book is intended for native and foreign consumption.

Wolfe, L. COOKING FOR THE CARIBBEAN ISLANDS. New York: Time-Life Books, 1970.

Background on the Caribbean Islands includes information on Cuba, Haiti, Dominican Republic, Jamaica, Puerto Rico, and many of the other 7,000 islands once known as the Antilles. Text is accompanied by recipes, most of which give country of origin. RECIPES: THE COOKING OF THE CARIBBEAN ISLANDS is the spiral bound volume of the recipes only.

Chapter 4

CHINESE AMERICANS

4.1 Introduction

The Chinese population has been growing rapidly since the 1960'6 when changes
in the immigration law took effect. Their origins vary, with some coming from
the People's Republic of China, others from Hong Kong or Taiwan (The Republic of China), and still others from dozens of smaller Asian nations, including
Korea, Vietnam, Laos, and Cambodia. Chinese cuisine may seem alike to those
unfamiliar with it but there are major differences, depending upon the cook's
country of origin, region of Chinese ancestry, ethnicity, and even whether there
was intermarriage from regions and groups within China and whether there has
been travel outside of China. These differences are very important, for the Chinese respect food, know and talk about it frequently, and share it often, it is one
of their greatest pleasures.

However, the Chinese do share a commonality, no matter what the internal
and external differences. The most important of these is called the "fan-tsai"
principle. "Fan" is the grain and "tsai" are the vegetables and other accompa-
niments of the meal. There is major north/south dichotomy within China of
the type of fan used. It is very important because the Chinese get about 80%
of their calories from grain. Those from south of the Yangtze River consume
rice; those north of it use wheat, millet, sorghum (kaoling), and some less well-
known and less popular grains though they, too, eat rice. The remaining 20%
of the calories are from vegetables, fruits, animal proteins, and fats. Another
universality, inculcated by Chinese parents, is that they leave the table 70% full.
There is, also, the concern for having a variety of textures, temperatures, and
tastes on every occasion that they share food. Chinese meals have a variety of
dishes to season the fan. An important cultural influence is the belief in "Yin"

65

and "Yang" or complementary forces that affect life. Foods and diseases are so labeled and one uses a "Yin" food to treat a "Yang" illness and a "Yang" food when the illness is considered "Yin."

The Chinese whether at home or abroad, usually eat three meals a day. For those of Southern heritage breakfast and lunch are similar, for those from the north lunch and dinner are much the same.

Southern breakfasts include "dim sum" or "dot the heart" items eaten in restaurants or tea houses morning and noon. The foods include dumplings steamed, fried, or baked. Literally hundreds may be available to choose from to "dot their hearts" and begin their day. These accompany "Congee," a rice gruel, that can be flavored with pickled vegetables, tiny bits of meat and/or legumes, nuts, or seeds. Northerners, for their breakfast, prefer soy milk and fried long crullers. These are dipped in sugar and then in warm or hot soy milk and eaten along with many pickled and stir-fried dishes.

Main meals contain rice or noodles and/or steamed bread along with several stir-fried, steamed or red-simmered dishes. Everyone gets a large bowl of the grain staple and chooses the accompanying tsai from common serving dishes. In Chinese cooking, all the food is cut up before it is cooked and served. It is eaten with chopsticks; no knives appear at the table. The use of chopsticks enables one to reach for tidbits from each of the accompanying dishes. There is no need to pass the dishes around the table.

Chinese do not eat desserts as familiar to westerners. Pastries are sometimes eaten with tea, more often they are reserved for special occasions and banquets. Beverages are different, too, for soup is the beverage of choice for 80% of the Chinese. Northerners like to drink the water their noodles have been cooked in, especially in winter. They drink it or soy milk, but the latter at breakfast only. Rarely do they drink tea at meals. The exception to this is that southerners take tea after or with their dim sum meals. Tea is always served to visitors, offered as a gesture of warmth and friendliness. Alcohol is rarely served, except to guests. The rare times that it is served, it is used for toasts at banquets and special meals.

In the past the Chinese rarely ate snacks. This is changing. Candy and bakery products are being consumed in increasing quantities and more frequently. These products were formerly reserved for children, guests, and holidays. Ice cream is popular and now part of the diet, but milk and milk products often are not. Manchurians and Tibetans use a limited quantity of dairy products, but most Chinese do not like them. They particularly dislike cheeses. Milk is acceptable for children; adults vary as to their consideration of its acceptability.

Overall, the diet is good. There is, however, some vitamin shortfall and concern about vitamin C, iron, and calcium. Caloric intake is related to economic considerations and a problem at the lower end. There is extensive use of sauces and all are high in sodium, oyster sauce having the least.

Problems occur as dietary patterns change. Recent research of immigrant populations shows rapid change of diet shortly after immigration and a return to more traditional food patterns after five or more years in the United States. No matter the duration of residence, Chinese prepare their foods Chinese-style, using locally available ingredients. Sharing is still considered the greatest of pleasures. Overall, many dislike dairy products and eat too many pickled and fermented products. Some incidence of cancer is attributed to this.

The Chinese get a large amount of their calories from polished rice and other highly milled grains and they eat more meat than ever before. They also wash their rice in many changes of water and rinse their noodles, too. While they do eat a quantity of vegetables, variety is limited and matches economic condition, less if money is short and greater with more affluence. They buy large sized fruits, but do not eat large quantities because each fruit is often shared at the table.

Lactose intolerance is amply reported in the literature, less about other food habits and beliefs or health related problems. This may be because the Chinese seek out traditional cures, including herbal remedies and acupuncture. They treat health as a personal problem and seek a doctor only as a measure of last resort.

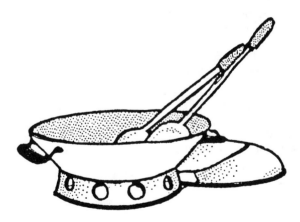

4.2   References

A BAREFOOT DOCTOR'S MANUAL. Philadelphia, PA: Running Press, 1977.

American translation of the official Chinese paramedical manual. Offers insight into acupuncture, massage, moxibustion, herbal preparations, diagnostic techniques, treatment of common diseases, hygiene, and birth control. The over 900 page-volume lists more than 190 diseases and 500 herbs. There are illustrations for about 300 herbs with uses and preparations for all. The text combines western and traditional Chinese practices and includes food prescriptions.

Anderson, E.N., and M.L. Anderson. "Cantonese ethnohoptology." ETHOS 1,4 (1969): 107-117.

Describes cooking typical of Cantonese and Hong Kong boat people. Includes meals, food symbolism and beliefs, and some social aspects of eating.

Bertino, M., G.K. Beauchamp, and K.C. Jen. "Rated taste perception in two culture groups." CHEM. SENSES 8 (1983): 3-15.

Intensity and pleasantness ratings of sucrose, caffeine and NaCl showed that Taiwanese students rated sucrose sweeter, and they rated low concentrations of NaCl as tasting saltier than did students of European descent born in the United States. There were no differences in the ratings of caffeine.

Campbell, T., and B. Chang. "Health care of the Chinese in America." NURS. OUTLOOK 21 (1973): 245-249.

Discusses problems of the hospitalized, general beliefs, food habits, nutrition, food and its relation to disease, and folk beliefs during pregnancy.

Carp, F.M., and E. Kataoka. "Health care problems of the elderly of San Francisco's Chinatown." GERONTOL. 16 (1976): 30-38.

Data on 138 elderly Chinese are from home interviews that include apperception pictures, food intake, and self-evaluations. Two-thirds rate their health as fair. Thirty percent indicate that health is their most serious problem and 43% visit a doctor or practitioner at least once a month.

Chan, D.W., and T.S.C. Chan. "Reliability, validity and the structure of the general health questionnaire in a Chinese context." PSYCHOL. MED. 13 (1983): 363-371.

Three questionnaires, the thirty-item General Health Questionnaire, 24-item Self-Reporting Questionnaire, and a Chinese version of the Minnesota Multiphasic Personality Inventory were administered to 225 English-speaking Chinese. The General Health Questionnaire is demonstrated to be psychometrically sound though the Chinese report more symptoms on withdrawal and depression than do Caucasians.

Chang, B. "Some dietary beliefs in Chinese folk culture." J. AMER. DIETET. ASSOC. 65 (1974): 436-438.

Article includes overview of yin/yang practices with foods and diseases, general food preferences, and special practices during child-bearing and post-partum periods.

Chang, C.C. CHIH KUEI YAO LUEH (PRESCRIPTIONS FROM THE GOLDEN CHAMBER). Long Beach, CA: Oriental Healing Arts Institute, 1983.

Translated into English by Wang Su-yen and Hsu Hong-yen, this centuries-old classic of Chinese medicine contains prescriptions for curing various diseases and conditions. Last two chapters discuss treatment of poisoning from eating meats, fish, fruits, vegetables, and cereals. Includes recipes for making the herbal prescriptions.

Chang, K.C., editor. FOOD IN CHINESE CULTURE. New Haven, CT: Yale University Press, 1977.

Book is a descriptive history of food habits in China from ancient times through Han, Tang, Sung, Yuan and Ming, and Ching dynasties into modern China, north and south. Nutritional, social, economic, and cosmological aspects are discussed; personal experiences are in the chapters on modern China. Includes significance of food making, food use, principal foodstuffs, methods for preparing and serving food, utensils, and customs of preparation and preserving, and their effects.

Chen, L.H., S.J. Hsu, P.C. Huang, and J.S. Chen. "Vitamin E status of Chinese population in Taiwan." AMER. J. CLIN. NUTR. 30 (1977): 728-735.

Data show plasma vitamin E levels with mean of 105mg/100ml. This is close to those of some groups but higher than others. The range in the 99 adults was 0.14 to 2.58mg/100ml with only seven percent deficient. There is no significant differences between sexes.

Cheng, T.O., B.B. Harrell, C.R. Dorso, R.I. Levin, A. Eldor, E.A. Jaffe, B.B. Weksler, and D.E. Hammerschmidt. "Chinese food and platelets." N. ENG. J. MED. 303 (1980): 756-757.

Letter makes reference to inhibition of platelet aggregation associated with eating Chinese cloud-ear mushrooms known as "mo-er" or black tree fungus. Related observations note need to be aware of interspecies differences in types of tree fungi. There is similar platelet effect with rootstock of ginger.

Cheung, L.Y.S., E.R. Cho, D. Lum, T.Y. Tang, and H.B. Yau. "The Chinese elderly and family structure: Implications for health care." PUBLIC HEALTH REP. 95 (1980): 491-495.

Data from 60 low-income elderly in California indicate most had immigrated less than 15 years before and 23% spoke very little English. Half had children nearby but the provision of support from them was marginal. They used a Chinese herbalist for minor illnesses and medical doctors for serious ones. The sample exhibited major psychological problems with respect to linguistic, economic, familial, and health issues.

Chew, D., B. So, and E. Bright-See. COUNSELING CHINESE PATIENTS. Toronto, Canada: The Canadian Diabetic Association, 1977.

Thirty-three page booklet on foods and uses, meal patterns, serving patterns and cultural beliefs. A glossary of Chinese foods and ingredients offers background.

Chew, T. "Sodium values of Chinese condiments and their use in sodium-restricted diets." J. AMER. DIETET. ASSOC. 82 (1983): 397-401.

Sodium content of 13 Chinese sauces and of dried shrimp are analyzed for sodium content by atomic absorption spectroscopy. Sweet bean, fermented black beans, hoisin, satay, fermented bean cake, and dried shrimp contained less than 200 mg. sodium per teaspoon. Variations did exist among brands. Soy sauce has the highest sodium content with light soy having more than dark. Oyster sauce has less than either of the soys with one brand of the latter only 213 mg/tsp.

Chinn, D. "Dietary beliefs and practices of the Chinese American elderly." M.S. thesis. California State University, 1977.

Most of the 25 elderly in this study have very little contact with the world outside of Chinatown. Income was generally around $2,000 per year, and housing poor for 28% of them. All preferred Chinese meals, 36% had a diet low in protein, 32% do not drink milk, and 25% lack adequate intake of vitamin C. Most are aware of both Chinese and western concepts of nutrition.

Chong, R., M. Holowaty, M. Krondl, and D. Lav. "The effect of culturally determined satiety meaning on food practices." J. CAN. DIETET. ASSOC. 37 (1976): 245-249.

Chinese and Ukrainians consider 36 food items and the effect of satiety meaning on food choice. Culture did affect choice but not frequency of use, satiety was not the dominant motive.

City of New York. FEEDING YOUR BABY. New York: Bureau of Nutrition, 1982.

Eight page bilingual Chinese and English pamphlet item discusses use of liquid and solid foods and daily meal plans in early and late infancy.

Czajkowski, J.M. CHINESE FOOD AND TRADITIONS. Storrs, CT: Connecticut Cooperative Extension Service, 1971.

Includes Chinese way with foods and the special foods they value, with recipes of typical dishes and meals. Describes food preparation and cooking methods and each page ends with a proverb.

Delendick, T.J., and S.K.M. Tim. PLANTS OF THE EARTH – THE CHINESE INFLUENCE. New York: Brooklyn Botanic Garden, 1980.

Discusses foods, fruits, spices and condiments, and medicinal plants in this 10-page booklet.

Dai, Y.T. "Iron fortification of Chinese soy sauce." FD. NUTR. BULL. 5 (1983): 35-52.

Studies show that ferrous sulfate in the amount of 75 to 100 mg has good solubility and would be good way to increase iron of one-third of the people of the world. Calculations show average Chinese uses 15 to 20 ml of soy sauce per day.

Gould-Martin, K. "Hot cold clean poison and dirt: Chinese folk medical categories." SOC. SCI. MED. 12 (1978): 39-46.

Discusses relationship between polarities of hot and cold, clean, poison, and dirt using fieldwork data. All of the categories are not opposites on a continuum, other relationships may exist.

Grivetti, L.E., and M.B. Paquette. "Non-traditional ethnic food choices among first generation Chinese in California." J. NUTR. EDUC. 10 (1978): 109-112.

Data from 30 Chinese interviewed show continued nonconsumption of certain foods in America despite availability. Seventy-seven foods investigated. Although pork, chicken, beef, and prawns were the animal products consumed most frequently in China, all but prawns still eaten often by more than 80%. Except for ice cream, diary products show low consumption. Rice remains the cereal of choice though its consumption declines after immigration. Vegetable use remains high with different vegetables used more in America, including broccoli, lettuce, potato, and squash. Fruit use increase is of apples and peaches and snack use changes.

HANDBOOK OF COMMONLY USED CHINESE HERBAL Prescription. Long Beach, CA: Oriental Healing Arts Institute, 1983.

Translated by Wang Yu-ching, this volume gives 210 Chinese herbal formulas approved by the Minstry of Health and Welfare of the Japanese government. Includes composition, form, dosage, origin, and indications for use.

Ho, Z.H. "Breast-feeding in Xinhui district in south China." FD. NUTR. BULL. 3,3 (1981): 42-48.

More than 99% of Chinese mothers breast feed, commonly up to one year, and 25% of infants 6 to 8 months old are not given any weaning foods. Describes dietary histories, anthropometric measurements, means of determining quantity of milk obtained from nursing, analysis of feeding and meal patterns, and home conditions.

Hou, X.C. "Egg preservation in China." FD. NUTR. BULL. 3,4 (1981): 17-20.

Four methods of preserving eggs with advise on coating ingredients, technique, and nutrients. Health claims for use include benefits for heart disease and high blood pressure. Studies of rats fed at 10% level show lowering of blood pressure and lipoprotein.

Hsia, P.Y.K., and D.L. Yeung. "A dietary study of adult Chinese-Canadians in Vancouver." CAN. J. 37 (1976): 164-172.

One-third of the 100 subjects speak English at the 24-hour dietary recall. Younger subjects are lower in height and weight than Canadians and overall the diet is inferior to that of the general Canadian population. Seventy-eight consume a continental breakfast, only 20% eat sandwiches, hamburgers, hot dogs, etc. for lunch, and at dinner Chinese food is the regular fare for all. Snacks contribute 7 to 13% of total calories and nutrients. Most calories and nutrients come from the evening meal. Of the nine dietary components examined, energy is least well supplied. Pork is the most frequently consumed meat, rice the most important grain. Milk and milk products are not used by the majority, and potatoes not eaten by most. Fruits are mostly apples and oranges.

Hsu, H.Y. HOW TO TREAT YOURSELF WITH CHINESE HERBS. Los Angeles, CA: Oriental Healing Arts Institute, 1980.

Designed as handbook of Chinese herbal medicine, book lists illnesses by category with several suitable herb combinations. Section on common herbs has Chinese and Latin names, specifics about the plant, uses, and often the principal chemical constituents. There is a treat yourself section and an appendix of herbs and their uses.

Hsu, H.Y., and W.G. Peacher. CHEN'S HISTORY OF CHINESE MEDICAL SCIENCE. Long Beach, CA: Oriental Healing Arts Institute, 1977.

This item originally published in Taiwan is English translation of Professor Chen Chan Yuen's HISTORY OF CHINESE MEDICAL SCIENCE ILLUSTRATED WITH PICTURES. It begins with Shen Nung the pharmacist of 3494 B.C. and goes through Wang Ching Jen, a well-known physiological anatomist who died in 1831, and Hsieh Li Heng, the 20th-century compiler of a medical dictionary. Refers to all the classic works through the centuries and ends with a chapter on the spread of Chinese medicine in Asia, to Europe and the United States.

Hsu., L.C. "Nutrition – from China to the West – art-science quality of nutrition." ECOL. FD. NUTR. 3 (1974): 303-314.

Shows, through commentary, the development and predominance of nutrition as an art in China. Criteria for and attitudes toward food and eating do not have quantitative and objective standards. Discusses why this might not work in the highly processed food system of the United States.

Hsu, L., and T.C. Tung. "Nutritional concepts and dietary practices in China." PROG. FD. NUTR. SCI. 2 (1977): 499-503.

Reviews current and historical nutrition concepts and present-day dietary practices in terms of what is eaten and how. Essential factors are choice of foods, importance of cutting and seasoning, and of proper service.

Huang, P.C., and C.P. Lin. "Protein requirements of young Chinese male adults on ordinary Chinese mixed diet and egg diet at ordinary levels of energy intake." J. NUTR. 112 (1982): 897-907.

Study of 28 males shows the digestibility of mixed and egg diet proteins was 96.5 and 98.0%, respectively. The efficiency of utilization of the Chinese mixed diet was 73 to 77% that of the egg protein diet, based on relative nitrogen requirements.

Huang, P.C., H.E. Chong, and W.M. Rand. "Obligatory urinary and fecal nitrogen losses in young Chinese men." J. NUTR. 102 (1972): 1605-1614.

Fifty healthy males ages 20 to 32 show obligatory urinary nitrogen normally distributed but in significantly lower amounts than Caucasian subjects. Statistically significant correlations among nitrogen and body weight, basal metabolic rate, and creatinine.

Hyatt, R. CHINESE HERBAL MEDICINE. New York: Schocken Books, 1978.

Offers introductory brief overview of history and traditions of herbal use. Sections on teas and other herbal preparations include amounts of individual ingredients, uses, and other conditions. Gives list of herbs most commonly used.

Jimenez, S.L.M. "Childhood in China." AMER. BABY 45,9 (1983): 26+.

Discusses traditional beliefs about childbirth, including shiatsu and acupuncture for easier pregnancy, and as currently practiced in China.

Jones, A.W. DOOR TO CHINESE FESTIVALS, FEASTS, FORTUNES. Taipei, Taiwan: Mei Ya Publications, 1971.

Describes Chinese New Year, Lantern, Dragon Boat, Ching Ming, and Moon festivals. Section on feasts gives more than 25 recipes with social, symbolic, and historical significances and section on fortunes introduces the Chinese zodiac or twelve-year cycle and gives the years of and fortunes for each.

Joos, S.K., E. Pollitt, and W.H. Mueller. "The Bacon Chow study: Effects of maternal nutritional supplement on infant mental and motor development." FD. NUTR. BULL. 4 (1982): 1-4.

Maternal nutritional supplementation during pregnancy and lactation have no effect on the Bayley mental-scale scores attained by infants at eight months of age. There is modest motor score gain of infants whose mothers take nutrition supplements. Findings are consistent with studies done in South America.

Kabes, S., A. Bailey, M. Brown, D. Clark, C.Y. Hsiao, and J. Miller. EX-PLORING THE PEOPLE'S REPUBLIC OF CHINA; NUTRITION AND ECOLOGY. St. Paul, MN: Minnesota Department of Education, n.d.

One of five units in Exploring the People's Republic of China series, others on arts, physical education, etc. Unit intended for junior/senior high schools is applicable to all ages; it includes maps, pictures, learning activities, and resource materials.

Kahn, E.J. "The staffs of life. IV – Everbody's business." THE NEW YORKER, March 4 1985, pp. 51-76.

Article is fourth in series of five, each on a major grain. This one on rice details current and historical information and its use in Asian and western countries.

Kerr, G.R., M. Wu-Lee, M. El-lozy, R. McGandy, and F.J. Stare. "Prevalence of the Chinese restaurant syndrome." J. AMER. DIETET. ASSOC. 75 (1975): 29-35.

Most of the 3,222 questionnaire respondents are aware of the syndrome and 43% experience unpleasant symptoms with specific foods and eating environments. One to two percent report symptoms considered characteristic of Chinese restaurant syndrome, and only 0.19% associate these with Chinese food.

Kleinman, A., P. Kunstadter, E.R. Alexander, and J.L. Gale, editors. MEDICINE IN CHINESE CULTURES: COMPARATIVE STUDIES OF HEALTH CARE IN CHINESE AND OTHER SOCIETIES. Washington, DC: U.S. Department of Health, Education, and Welfare, 1975.

Most of the 49 chapters relate to Chinese generally or to those in China, Taiwan, or Hong Kong. The others concern those in Burma, Malaysia, India, Sri Lanka, and the rest of Asia. All represent a broad range of disciplines including medical, anthropological, historical, etc. Book is more than 800 pages long and contains detailed references at the end of each chapter.

Koh, T.H.H.G. "Breast feeding among Chinese in four countries." J. TROP. PEDIATRICS 27,2 (1981): 88-91.

Discusses Chinese women in Malay, Singapore, China, and Britain. In Malay and China virtually all babies are breast fed, in Singapore more poor mothers breast feed than do well-to-do and do so longer than the affluent mothers. In Glasgow, only two percent of the Chinese babies are breast fed.

Koo, L.C.L. NOURISHMENT OF LIFE. Hong Kong: The Commercial Press, 1982.

Book discusses health in a Chinese society. The importance of body image, sex, physical therapy, spiritual and emotional health, and diet and food are covered. Report includes seven-day dietary surveys and 500-item food classification surveys on hot/cold, wet, clashing, poisonous, or nourishing characteristics. While concentrating on populations in Taiwan and San Francisco the results and information can be generalized to include Chinese worldwide.

Koo, L.C. "Traditional Chinese diet and its relationship to health." KROEBER ANTHRO. SOC. PAPERS 47-48 (1973): 116-147.

Holistic analysis of Chinese food habits shows diet related to social organization, land use, beliefs, maintenance of health, and demographics. Typical and holiday meals, sources of protein, delicacies, preparation and cookery, nutritional evaluation of Chinese diets, and hot and cold theory are explored. Includes list of hot, cold, neutral, poisonous, and nutritious foods.

Koo, L.C. "The use of food to treat and prevent disease in Chinese culture." SOC. SCI. MED. 18,9 (1984): 757-766.

Interviews with 50 families in Hong Kong indicate that food is the most important method of dealing with the prevention and treatment of 59 common symptoms and illnesses. Selection, timing, and preparation of the food is of concern. Food prescriptions are based on traditional yin/yang qualities of body energy or chi. Dietary management of disease complements western medicine and is predominant at the beginning and end of pathogenesis.

Lee, R.P.L. "Perceptions and uses of Chinese medicine among the Chinese in Hong Kong." CULT. MED. PSYCH. 4 (1980): 345-375.

Findings from several studies and from qualitative observations suggest that about 20% follow magical-religious traditions of Chinese medicine, over 50% use secular medicine, and most are more confident in the Chinese medical tradition than in western medicine. The process of medical care is a pattern of self-medication, use of Chinese or western home remedies, western style doctors, Chinese style practitioners, and finally a western medical hospital.

Li, F.P., N.Y. Schlief, C.J. Chang, and A.C. Gaw. "Health care for the Chinese community in Boston." AMER. J. PUB. HEALTH 62 (1972): 536-539.

Reports on the efforts of one community to affect the health of the Chinese community by coordinating existing health facilities. Surveyed 200 households to assess their use and learned that 20% were unaware of their existence, only 25% could speak English, and 50% admitted self medication with herbs.

Ling, S., J. King, and V. Leung. "Diet, growth, and cultural food habits in Chinese American infants." AMER. J. CHINESE MED. 3,2 (1975): 125-132.

One hundred Chinese American mothers and infants studied have infant growth patterns dissimilar to those of infants in China or the United States. They are, however, similar to growth patterns in underdeveloped countries. In general, cultural beliefs are adhered to, 47% of the mothers eat one or more herbs during pregnancy, and 53% follow traditional taboos during that time. About one-fourth of the infants are fed some sort of Chinese herb.

Ludman, E.K., and J.M. Newman. "Yin and yang in health related food practices of three Chinese groups." J. NUTR. EDUC. 16 (1984): 3-5.

Discusses relationship of yin and yang to diet therapy in 394 respondents from China, Hong Kong, and the United States. They indicate that food and herb therapy continues to affect their dietary practices and yin and yang diet therapy is practiced. Eighty-seven percent of the Chinese dealing with fever, 60% with pregnancy, and 74% with blood building say they use special foods as treatment. Tables include yin/yang foods and diseases.

Luo, X, H. Wei, C. Yang, J. Xing, C. Qiao, Y. Feng, J. Liu, Z. Liu, Q. Wu, Y. Liu, B.S. Stoecker, J.E. Spallholz, and S.P. Yang. "Selenium intake and metabolic balance of 10 men from a low selenium area of China." AMER. J. CLIN. NUTR. 42 (1985): 31-37.

Self-selected diets of ten healthy men show selenium intake at 8.8 micrograms per day, well below that recommended. Apparent absorption is approximately 57%.

Missine, L.E. "Elders are educators." PERSPEC. AGING (November/December 1982): 5-8.

View of aging in China shows continuation of respect, authority, and usefulness in society. Childless elderly guaranteed food, clothing, shelter, medical care, and burial.

Newman, J.M. "Bakery products of China." CER. FD. WORLD 26 (1981): 395-399.

Bakery products and moon cakes have about same caloric value as American cookies per 100 grams, but as Chinese items are heavier, intake is higher. Nutrient content of eight items included.

Newman, J.M. "Chinese American food: Diet of the future?" J. HOME ECON. 68,5 (1976): 39-43.

Reviews traditional meals, snacks, breakfasts, protein foods, other food groups, beverages, and sauces. Implications for better United States nutrition given.

Newman, J.M., and R. Linke. "Chinese immigrant food habits: A study of the nature and direction of change." ROYAL SOC. HEALTH J. (London) 102,6 (1982): 268-271.

Study researches 102 immigrants to Queens and Chinatown in New York City, using questionnaires and interviews. Significant changes of food habits occur immediately after immigration, though less for those in Chinatown. After more than five years in the United States there is a reversal to some traditional food habits no matter where the people live. The most significant changes are for meats and dairy items.

Newman, J.M., and E.K. Ludman. "Chinese elderly: Food habits and beliefs." J. NUTR. ELDERLY 4,2 (1984): 3-13.

Comparison of Chinese elderly in China and the United States reveals more striking similarities than differences. Data show that traditional beliefs still control dietary practices. Over 90% drink soup as the beverage of choice at meals, 27% tea, and 20% water. No other beverage is consumed by more than 10%. Fifty-eight percent buy special foods for the elderly and about half of these are high in protein.

Newman, J.M., Contento, I., and Kris. E. "Perspectives on food and nutrition in the People's Republic of China." J. NUTR. EDUC. 13 (1981): 43-45.

Overviews food and its distribution, nutrition research, and public health in China, listing individuals and institutions.

Pillsbury, B.L.K. "'Doing the month': Confinement and convalescence of Chinese women after childbirth." SOC. SCI. MED. 12 (1978): 11-22.

One hundred percent of more than 100 Chinese and Chinese Americans interviewed considered "doing the month" efficacious for physical health or social relations. This included refraining from washing and all contact with water and wind, use of a "hot" diet to remedy hot/cold imbalance, and observing other taboos.

Quinn, J.R., editor. CHINA MEDICINE AS WE SAW IT. Washington, DC: Department of Health, Education, and Welfare, 1974.

Book offers views of acupuncture, fractures, limb reattachment, public health organization and practices, and biomedical research.

Rainey, C. CHINESE CUISINE. Columbia, MO: University of Missouri-Columbia, 1977.

Packet includes maps, pictures, food patterns, nutrition and food habits, food preparation, meal service information, activities, games, and background materials.

Schreiver, L., editor. HEALTH IS WEALTH. New York: Chinatown Planning Council, n.d.

A Chinese patient handbook written in Chinese and English with sections on medical history, directions, emergencies, medical problems, staff questions and instructions to patients, medication instructions, appointments, hospital and clinic information, and rights as a patient. Also has directory of hospitals and clinics in New York City in this small and easy to carry booklet.

Sly, T., and E. Ross. "Chinese foods: Relationship between hygiene and bacterial flora. J. FD. PROTEC. 45 (1982): 115-124.

Commercial meals in restaurants in Ontario, Canada, are examined. Bacillus cereus isolated in nine percent of the 116 samples. No Salmonella or Clostridium perfringens found.

Snapper, I. CHINESE LESSONS TO WESTERN MEDICINE. New York: Grune and Stratton, 1965.

This second edition of a 1941 volume updates the earlier one and has chapter on nutritional problems and avitaminosis, B_1 deficiency in heart failure, cardiovascular diseases, and other medical issues.

So, B., D. Chew, and E. Bright-See. "Dietetic counseling of Chinese diabetic patients." J. CAN. DIETET. ASSOC. 39,1 (1978): 46-53.

Article reports survey of 25 hospitals for their exchange lists for Chinese diabetic patients. Availability of booklets prepared for counseling and 166 slides of traditional Chinese foods and herbs to aid recognition by non-Chinese counselors mentioned. Tables of foods include exchange lists, free foods, foods to use occasionally with their exchanges, and foods to avoid.

Soong, F.S. "Beliefs and practices of Chinese diabetic patients concerning the cause and treatment of their ill-health." SING. MED. J. 12 (1971): 309-313.

Finds 68% used Chinese medicines in addition to western-style treatments. Only 4% knew the true cause of diabetes and 74% understood that treatment cannot affect a radical cure. Of those using non-western therapeutic measures, twice as many females as males took home remedies (64%), 24% bought medicines from Chinese stores, 30% used advice of Sinsehs, and 10% used advice of Tangki. The responses show use of more than one source.

Tan, S.P., and E. Wheeler. "Changing dietary patterns among Hong Kong Chinese families now settled in London." NUTR. SOC. PRO. 41 (1982): 45A.

Longitudinal study of 31 families visited on four occasions shows dietary pattern is based on what would be eaten in Hong Kong, especially for the evening meal. Convenience foods enter the diet for breakfast. Mothers think school meal is not very nourishing; they supplement it after school with cold drinks, bread, Chinese snack foods and cakes, and/or special herbal drinks.

Terashi, B. THE PROBLEMS OF AGING. Long Beach, CA: Oriental Healing Arts Institute, 1984.

Discusses heart and circulatory, respiratory, gastrointestinal, liver, kidney, genital, gynecological, skin, metabolic, and mental disorders in terms of western and Chinese treatment. Each is followed by herbal combinations and their specific uses. The appendix lists ingredients in the herbal formulas. The text offers some case studies by a doctor of western and Chinese medicine.

Townshend, J.R. THE PEOPLE'S REPUBLIC OF CHINA. New York: China Council of the Asia Society and the Council on International and Public Affairs, 1979.

A basic handbook on the land and its people with some history, government, and economic information, and sections on social organization, education, public health, and daily life. Reference section includes sources for books, bibliographies, current events, teachers' materials, and guides for the traveler.

Tseng, R.Y.L., E. Smith-Nury, and Y.S. Chang. "Calcium and phosphorus contents and ratios in tofu as affected by the coagulents used." HOME ECON. RES. J. 6 (1977): 171-175.

Analysis of three commercial brands of tofu shows that the firm tofu precipitated with calcium sulfate contains over four times as much calcium and over twice the phosphorus as soft tofu made with glucono delta lactone.

United States Department of Education. BIBLIOGRAPHY. Kansas City, MO: Region VII Refugees Materials Center, 1983.

Materials are for many ethnic groups, one section is for Chinese-speaking refugees. It includes extensive list of available cultural materials, guide for taking medicine, catalog of health education materials, etc., in English and/or Chinese.

Wallnofer, H., and A.V. Rottauscher. CHINESE FOLK MEDICINE. New York: Bell Publishing Co., 1965.

Translated by Marion Palmedo, this volume has treatments and alleged cures that have been in use for centuries. They appear after introduction of fundamentals of Chinese medicine and the age old philosophy from which it originates. Sections include anatomy, physiology, pathology, pulse theory, various treatment methods, material on aging and dying, cosmetics, and dreams and their interpretation. Book is by medical doctor and a colleague who have utilized and synthesized the oldest Chinese texts on these subjects.

Wang, M., and J.T. Dwyer. "Reaching Chinese American children with nutrition education." J. NUTR. EDUC. 7 (1975): 145-148.

Suggests that supplemental culture-specific classroom instruction enhances the effect of film instruction and other types of materials. For instruction to be meaningful, illustrative materials must show oriental subjects.

Wen, C.P. "Food and Nutrition in the People's Republic of China." CHINA MEDICINE AS WE SAW IT. Edited by J.R. Quinn. Washington, DC: U.S. Department of Health, Education, and Welfare, 1974, pp. 181-246.

Nutritional epidemiologist discusses improvement of Chinese diet, role food plays in nutriture, clinicophysical evaluations, medical status, international comparisons, and other health information.

Whang, J. "Chinese traditional food therapy." J. AMER. DIETET. ASSOC. 78 (1981): 55-57.

Explains that ancient Chinese medical practices emphasize dietary factors in prevention and cure diseases and maintenance of health through food therapy. Prevention, cure, and nourishment are highlighted, as are taboos and their relation to disease. Some hot and cold foods and related disease use is given as an illustration of the need to consider ancient beliefs for maximum effectiveness in diet therapy.

Wheeler, E., and T.S. Poh. "Food for equilibrium: The dietary principles and practice of Chinese families in London." In THE SOCIOLOGY OF FOOD AND EATING. Edited by A. Murcott. Hants, England: Gower Publishing Co., 1983, pp.84-94.

In fifty families all but one have females practicing a pragmatic version of traditional medicine and health care with their choice of foods influenced by this system. Their teen-agers are not learning the system in depth as they used to.

Wheeler, E., and S.P. Tan. "From concept to practice: Food behavior of Chinese immigrants in London." ECOL FD. NUTR. 13 (1983): 51-57.

Dietary practices of 50 families from Hong Kong describe their conceptualization. Pattern of consumption is varied and nutritionally excellent with little incorporation of English food. Foods eaten at various stages of the life cycle are described as are their cultural meanings.

World Bank. CHINA. Volume III: THE SOCIAL SECTORS POPULATION, HEALTH, NUTRITION, AND EDUCATION. Washington, DC: The World Bank, 1980.

Overview in hundreds of pages and dozens of charts what is happening in China with special emphasis on health and nutrition. Valuable as background material for understanding modern China and the Chinese.

Wu, F.Y.T. "Mandarin-speaking aged Chinese in the Los Angeles area." GERONTOL. 15 (1975): 271-275.

Describes relationships and adjustments of the elderly, including their having to endure many changes from filial piety to politics.

Yang, G.I.P., and H. Fox. "Food habit changes of Chinese persons living in Lincoln, Nebraska." J. AMER. DIETET. ASSOC. 75 (1979): 420-424.

Study of qualitative and quantitative changes in food habits of first-generation Chinese shows incorporation of American foods prepared in a Chinese manner. Some decrease in use of Chinese foods and a flexible attitude are shown. American food is used at breakfast and lunch; at dinner Chinese foods are preferred.

Yeung, D.L., L.W.Y. Cheung, and J.H. Sabry. "The hot-cold concept in Chinese culture and its application in a Chinese-Canadian community." CAN. DIETET. ASSOC. J. 34 (1973): 197-203, 209.

Fifty households respond to a questionnaire for an interview, many others do not. Chinese meals are served at least once each day in 78% of the households, two-thirds have family members eating every meal together. Responses indicate hot-cold concepts are well accepted but majority of the respondents unable to define them in simple terms. Ninety-two percent describe symptoms believed due to excess of hot foods, 75% say they avoid hot foods if they have these symptoms.

Yin, P., and K.W. Lai. "A reconceptualization of age stratification in China." J. GERONTOL. 38 (1983): 608-613.

Research suggests no change in age stratification as evaluated from the literature. Rather, there seems to be an increase in status.

Zheng, J.J., and I.H. Rosenberg. "Lactose malabsorption in healthy Chinese adults." ECOL. FD. NUTR. 15 (1984): 1-6.

Hydrogen breath tests reveal that 75% of the 20 subjects demonstrate malabsorption of 25 grams of lactose and 86.7% of these experience gastrointestinal symptoms during the test. Symptoms occur one half to two hours after ingestion; these usually last for four hours.

4.3   Resources for Recipes

Chang, I.B., W.W. Chang, A.H. Kutscher, and H.W. Kutscher. AN ENCY-
CLOPEDIA OF CHINESE FOOD AND COOKING. New York: Crown
Publishers, 1970.

More than 1,000 recipes, each indicating region of origin. Volume has detailed background information and an extensive glossary of ingredients that includes type, shape, color, surface, consistency, aroma, taste, available forms,
storage, substitution. Recipes in food category chapters have ingredients as-
signed letters of the alphabet, these letters are then used in explanations of
preparation and cooking techniques.

Chao, B.Y. HOW TO COOK AND EAT IN CHINESE. New York: John
Day Co., 1945.

Classic early volume that is reprinted frequently in paperback. Introductory
section is frequently quoted for preparation, cooking, and eating methods and
materials. Recipes are from all regions but do not so indicate. They are in food
category chapters. Throughout there are helpful hints, food habits, and folkloric
information.

Chu, G.Z. MADAME CHU'S CHINESE COOKING SCHOOL. New York:
Simon and Schuster, 1975.

More than 200 recipes tested in classes, with answers to questions often
posed by students. There are an introduction on the regions of China and
cooking techniques and a section with recipes contributed by students. The
volume ends with a glossary of dozens of ingredients, each with its name in large
size ideographs.

Chu, G.Z. THE PLEASURES OF CHINESE COOKING. New York: Simon
and Schuster, 1962.

Early classic has recipes grouped according to difficulties of obtaining ingredients and preparation. Introductory section has ingredient information, preparation and cooking materials, the story of tea, restaurant ordering advice, even
growing one's own beansprouts. The book also has sections on banquet dishes,
dim sum, and four regional ways to prepare duck.

Claiborne, C., and V. Lee. THE CHINESE COOKBOOK. New York: Lippincott Co., 1972.

Detailed introduction of equipment, methods, and tips is followed by over 240 recipes from varied regions, not so indicated, in chapters titled by food categories. A glossary of ingredients that includes some storage information has large ideographs. Recipes are authentic, detailed, and easy to follow.

Dahlen, M., and K. Phillipps. A POPULAR GUIDE TO CHINESE VEG-
ETABLES. New York: Crown Publishers, 1983.

Common, typically Chinese vegetables are illustrated in color, usually one to a page with details on appearance, quality, preparation, cooking, and other general commentary. Some have a recipe typical of the item. Appendix lists botanical and English names, Cantonese pronunciation, and Chinese ideographs.

Fu, P.M. PEI MEI'S CHINESE COOK BOOK. Taipei, Taiwan: n.p., 1969.

The author is the Julia Child of Taiwan. This is the first of three volumes, all reprinted many times, with recipes in Chinese and English, one to a page. This volume has dishes in three regional designations: Eastern, Southern, and Northern, and a fourth section on snacks and desserts. Photographs of some of the dishes appear before each section. Volume II is divided into chapters by food category and Volume III contains nine formal banquet dinners from different provinces; Taiwanese, vegetarian, and buffet dinners are included.

Hahn, E., editor. THE COOKING OF CHINA. New York: Time-Life Books,
1968.

One of the volumes in the Foods of the World series with introduction on history of the cuisine and chapters on seasoning, cooking, concerns for good food, rice, teas, festivals, and cooking Chinese food outside of China. Recipes appear throughout and also in a separate volume with no background or text.

Huang, H.Y. HOW TO COOK CHINESE VEGETARIAN DISHES. Taipei,
Taiwan: Tang's Publishing Co., 1979.

While some recipes have animal names, all are made from only vegetable ingredients. Each appears in English and in Chinese, has values given for ten nutrients, and has a color photograph of the completed dish. An explanation and method of making special ingredients appear at the end of the book.

Huang, S.H. CHINESE CUISINE. Taipei, Taiwan: School of Home Economics of the Wei-Chuan Foods Co., 1972.

Recipes by food category follow a color photograph of commonly used vegetables and another of dry materials. All recipes indicate region of origin and

have a color photograph of the completed dish, one to a page. Other volumes; CHINESE SNACKS, CHINESE APPETIZERS AND GARNISHES, and CHINESE COOKING FOR BEGINNERS, are also available.

Kan, L. INTRODUCING CHINESE CASSEROLE COOKERY. New York: Workman Publishing Co., Inc., 1978.

Family style one-pot stews, braised dishes, and combination pots from many culinary regions are listed by main ingredient and follow some preparation techniques.

Lee, B. THE EASY WAY TO CHINESE COOKING. New York: Dolphin Books, 1963.

Basic information on ingredients, their uses and storage, and details on preparation and cooking methods. Recipes are divided into chapters by cooking method and include descriptions of chow or stir-frying, jing or steaming, and red cooking. There are others on rice and noodle dishes, soups, wines and teas, and desserts.

Leung, M. THE CLASSIC CHINESE COOK BOOK. New York: Harper & Row, 1976.

Recipes from six provinces are detailed in an easy-to-follow manner, without compromising authenticity. A running commentary offers history, habit, and heritage. The glossary of cooking ingredients details purchase, use, and storage instructions.

Lin, F. FLORENCE LIN'S VEGETARIAN COOKBOOK. New York: Hawthorn Books, 1976.

This is a guide to the Chinese way of cooking vegetables, soybeans and soy products, other legumes, wheat gluten, eggs, seeds and nuts, and various grains, including rice and wheat. There is a detailed glossary of Chinese ingredients with purchase, use, and storage information. This is one of several by this author.

Lin, H.J., and T. Lin. CHINESE GASTRONOMY. New York: Hastings House Publishers, 1969.

This is an often quoted volume that combines history, classic and home cuisine, and other background information. Illustrative recipes are in chapters on ancient cuisine, flavor, texture, regional cooking, curiosities, plain and classic cooking, and a gastronomic calendar.

Liu, C.Y.C. NUTRITION AND DIET WITH CHINESE COOKING. Ann Arbor, MI: By the author, 1977.

Introductory section on nutrition, customs, preparation, utensils, and menu planning precedes the recipes listed by food category. Each recipe lists calories, protein, carbohydrate, and fat content. There is a short ingredient list with explanations and a few charts that are nutrition related.

Lo, E.Y. THE DIM SUM BOOK. New York: Crown Publishers, 1982.

Dim sum are traditional teahouse foods; they include dumplings, congees, cakes, rolls, and other "dot the heart" small items. Recipes for these follow detailed information on ingredients, techniques, and equipment. Line drawings illustrate their traditional shapes.

Lo, K. A GUIDE TO CHINESE EATING. Oxford, England: Phaidon Press, 1976.

This volume by this very prolific Chinese born English cookbook author explains the cuisine. It does so by offering extensive introductory information and describing about 100 dishes with regard to taste, appearance, and ingredients. Dishes and terms are given in Mandarin and Cantonese transliterations.

Lo, K. NEW CHINESE COOKING SCHOOL. Tuscon, AZ: HP Books, 1985.

Extensive list of equipment, glossary of food terms, and recipes, each giving level of difficulty, cooking method, serving size, and cooking time.

Ma, N.C. MRS. MA'S CHINESE COOKBOOK. Rutland, VT: Charles E. Tuttle Co., 1960.

One of many books by this international authority, it includes basic background information, recipes divided by season, and chapters on rice, noodles, dumplings, and desserts. There is some basic information on table setting, service, and behavior.

Miller, G.B. THE THOUSAND RECIPE CHINESE COOKBOOK. New York: Atheneum, 1966.

Recipes adapted for Americans with many variations for most of them. They follow a very detailed introductory section on history, regions, ingredients, techniques, equipment, and basics. The third part, entitled Supplementary Information, could be a valuable book in its own right. It includes preparing, setting, serving, and menu suggestions and the most detailed information on ingredients, substitutions, storing, and soaking.

Perkins, D.W., editor. HONG KONG CHINA AND GAS COOKBOOK. Hong Kong: Pat Printer Associates, 1978.

A beautifully produced and lavishly illustrated volume that offers more than 100 pages of detailed background information of history, ingredients, equipment, preparation, and cooking materials. Recipes follow as does a section on eating and drinking, and a glossary of ingredients with purchase and storage information.

Sakanoto, N. THE PEOPLE'S REPUBLIC OF CHINA COOKBOOK. New York: Random House, 1977.

More than 200 recipes originally published in cookbooks in China are presented after an introduction on utensils, cutting, and cooking methods. The recipes are divided into sections denoted by compass points N, E, SE, and SW.

Schrecker, E., with J. Schrecker. MRS. CHIANG'S SZECHWAN COOKBOOK. New York: Harper & Row, Publishers, 1976.

Offers introductory information on the spirit of the cuisine, banquet and home cooking differences, the regional cuisines, ingredients, equipment, methods, and menu planning. This is followed by recipes of the southwestern province of Szechwan divided into food category chapters.

Simonds, N. CLASSIC CHINESE CUISINE. Boston: Houghton Mifflin Co., 1983.

This volume by the author of 24 monthly articles in GOURMET MAGAZINE includes background materials, a glossary, and classic recipes with some culinary and cultural lore. The recipes are divided by food category, are clearly written, and easy to follow.

Chapter 5

JAPANESE AMERICANS

5.1 Introduction

Japanese food and food habits stand apart because of the special concern for simplicity, purity, and beauty. All foods are meticulously prepared; extreme refinement in presentation is important at the Japanese table.

The Japanese prize individual ingredients. They do not blend herbs and spices; there are very few instances offering bouquets of flavors. They offer compositions on the plate, not in the pot. Most of their foods are prepared quickly. There are some external influences that have broadened their early diet of fish, seaweed, vegetables, and fruit. The first were from their Chinese neighbors and later the influences were broadened by contacts with Portuguese from Macao. Western influences came much later still, after the Second World War.

Japanese meals are light, have limited use of animal fat, and little starch except for rice. Flavorings are mild, long cooking rare, and pickled vegetables ubiquitous. Meals contain fish, vegetables – pickled, fresh, or both, other pickled items, soup, and tea. Soybean products are present as miso (the soup), tofu (beancurd), and/or shoyu (soy sauce). A light dessert such as fruit juice, jelly, or iced bean curd may be served. Western style desserts are rare. The food is served on lacquered trays and eaten with chop sticks. The presentation of the food is artistic and beautiful and is in harmony with the season and with the dishes upon which each item is served.

Meats are becoming more popular in Japan as they are with Japanese in the United States. They are served in addition to or in place of the fish or seafood. Milk is becoming more popular but it is not an important part of the diet; the Japanese and other Asians get their calcium and phosphorus by eating dark green vegetables and tender fish bones. Unlike their Chinese neighbors, the Japanese do eat salads and other raw foods and they do so either before or after their main course. Rice is eaten in the traditional way and as rice noodles. It is not the only grain; many noodles are also consumed made from buckwheat or wheat. These are served hot in soups or cold as a salad.

The Japanese are not eaters of sweets but they do use a lot od sugar as seasoning. Even their soy sauce is sweet, sweeter than the soy sauces of the Chinese. Tea accompanies meals. Sake is a sweet wine and it accompanies traditional, guest, and restaurant dinners. In addition, tea is used alone as a snack food or with light dessert items. Japanese tea may be made from tea leaves, from barley, or from toasted wheat grains.

Breakfast for the Japanese is frequently a hot bowl of rice gruel or "congee" or it is a soup made from fermented bean paste. Lunch or dinner is as indicated above. Families serve all foods at once, not in course order at their meals. Eating patterns are changing with adoption of American foods and food habits, meals are now higher in meats, fats, and total calories and lower in the use of vegetables. The use of pickled vegetables has remained constant. Its use and the use of fermented food items are of concern in both Japan and in the United States as is the concern about the increasing consumption of fats and total calories. Increases in hypertension and reports of some stomach and intestinal cancers have been reported.

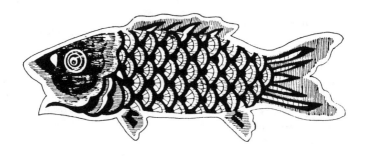

5.2 References

Abaika, M.H. "Japanese American food equivalents for calculating Exchange diets." J. AMER. DIETET. ASSOC. 62 (1973): 173-180.

Explains Japanese food patterns and why it is important to understand them. Describes typical foods and discusses nutrient content and carbohydrate, protein, fat, and energy exchanges. Includes some data on the sodium and potassium content of foods high in these minerals.

Finegold, S.M., H.R. Attebery, and V.L. Sutter. "Effect of diet on human fecal flora: Comparison of Japanese and American diets." AMER. J. CLIN. NUTR. 27 (1974): 1456-1459.

Finds extremely oxygen sensitive anaerobes more common in the Japanese diet than in the western diet through study of fecal flora of the 33 subjects, fifteen of whom were primarily on a Japanese diet. Americans have lower amounts of clostridium in their stool. Finds more than 220 distinct groups of bacteria of those on Japanese diet, more than 160 of those on the American diet.

Haenszel, W., M. Kurihara, M. Segi, and R.K.C. Lee. "Stomach cancer among Japanese in Hawaii." J. NATL. CANCER INST. 49 (1972): 969-988.

Study of 220 Japanese patients with stomach cancer and 440 controls reveals that those from regions with the highest stomach cancer risks in Japan continue to display an excess risk after migration to Hawaii. This does not persist among their offspring.

Hankin, J.H., A. Nomura, and G.G. Rhoads. "Patterns among men of Japanese ancestry in Hawaii." CANCER RES. 35 (1975): 3259-3264.

The dietary pattern of 6,663 men of Japanese ancestry participating in the Honolulu Heart and Japan-Hawaii Cancer studies finds the second generation eating lesser quantities of typically Japanese foods and their total intake of animal protein, total and saturated fat, and cholesterol significantly higher.

Higashi, A., T. Ikeda, I. Uehara, and I. Matsuda. "Zinc and copper contents in breast milk of Japanese women." TOHOKU J. EXPER. MED. 137 (1982): 41-46.

Evaluates breast milk of 65 mothers to five months postpartum. Finds the highest levels of zinc in the colostrum with levels declining as lactation progresses. Copper levels remain steady in first month, then they, too, decline.

Insull, W., Jr., T. Oiso, and K. Tsuchiya. "Diet and nutritional status of Japanese." AMER. J. CLIN. NUTR. 21 (1968): 753-777.

Describes current food intake, daily intake in food categories and individual items, and current nutritional status. Discusses these in terms of the carefully documented national statistics for the preceding 20 years. Bibiliography is of Japanese and American research and is extensive.

Kagan, A., B.R. Harris, W. Winkelstein, Jr., K.G. Johnson, H. Kat, S.L. Syme, G.H. Rhoads, M.L. Gay, M.Z. Nichaman, H.B. Hamilton, and J. Tillotson. "Epidemiologic studies of coronary heart disease and stroke in Japanese men living in Japan, Hawaii, and California: Demographic, physical, dietary, and biochemical characteristics." J. CHRON. DIS. 27 (1974): 345-364.

The study of thousands of subjects in each of the three countries indicate weights of Californians (C) heavier than those in Hawaii (H) and these heavier than those in Japan (J). Blood pressures from highest to lowest are C, H, J, cholesterol ranges in the same order, likewise means of uric acid. Some similarities exist between C and H. Proportion of calories from diet follows the same pattern for protein and fat, with the reverse order for carbohydrates and alcohol.

Kagawa, Y. "Impact of westernization on the nutrition of the Japanese: Changes in physique, cancer, longevity, and centarians." PREV. MED. 7 (1978): 205-217.

Traditional diet in years 1950 to 1975 shows 15-fold increase for milk, 7.5 for meat, poultry, and six fold for eggs. Barley use is only one-fortieth, potato use is down 50% and rice consumption down 0.7%. During this period, Japanese are taller and heavier. Breast, colon, and lung cancers increase two to three times, while those of the stomach and uterus decrease. Life expectancy is extended 12 years for males, 14 for females.

Kanada, H., K. Tobinai, J. Matsumoto, T. Maeta, T. Murata, T. Haruyama, and M. Imawari. "Effect of vitamin D_2 on hypocalcemia under chronic hemodialysis." TOHOKU J. EXPER. MED. 131 (1980): 249-256.

Bone lesions and hypocalcemia are treatable with vitamin D_3 in patients with chronic renal failure. Use of vitamin D_2 is appropriate and suitable dose may be related to duration of dialysis. Effects of vitamin D_2 on hypocalcemia in dialyzed patients partly dependent on the residual renal function with respect to conversion of $25\text{-}OH\text{-}D_3$ into $1,25\text{-}OH_2D_3$.

Kawasaki, T., M. Ueno, K. Uezono, M. Matsuoka, T. Omae, F. Halberg, H. Wendt, M.A. Taggett-Anderson, and E. Haus. "Differences and similarities among circadian characteristics of plasma renin activity in healthy young women in Japan and the United States." AMER. J. MED. 68 (1980): 91-96.

Blood sample analysis reveals urinary excretion of sodium and chloride statistically different and contributing to lower mesor values in women from Japan; this difference attributed to dietary salt.

Kawate, R., M. Yamakido, Y. Nishimoto, P.H. Bennett, R.F. Hamman, and W.C. Knowler. "Diabetes mellitus and its vascular complications in Japanese migrants on the island of Hawaii." DIABETES CARE 2 (1979): 161-200.

Proportion of deaths attributed to diabetes is much higher in Japanese migrants than in those living in Japan though caloric intake is similar. Consumption of animal fat is twice as high for Japanese in Hawaii as those in Japan, as is consumption of simple carbohydrates.

Kishi, K., S. Miyatani, and G. Inoue. "Requirement and utilization of egg protein by Japanese young men with marginal intakes of energy." J. NUTR. 108 (1978): 658-669.

Marginal intakes of energy are evaluated in 46 men; their nitrogen and NPU balance are affected by energy intake and the NPU for egg protein was about 50 to 55.

Kolonel, L.N., A.M.Y. Nomura, T. Hirohata, J.H. Hankin, and M.W. Hinds. "Association of diet and place of birth with stomach cancer incidence in Hawaii Japanese and Caucasians." AMER. J. CLIN. NUTR. 34 (1981): 2478-2485.

Japanese migrants to Hawaii have higher age-adjusted incidence of stomach cancer than Japanese born in Hawaii. Caucasian migrants to Hawaii, chiefly from the continental United States, have lower rates than Caucasians born in Hawaii. Dietary data reveal positive associations of stomach cancer with rice, pickled vegetables, and dried and/or salted fish and negative associations with consumption of ascorbic acid.

Marmot, M.G., and S.L. Syme. "Acculturation and coronary heart disease in Japanese Americans." AMER. J. EPIDEMIOL. 104 (1976): 225-247.

Explores role of social and cultural differences in incidence of coronary heart disease among 3,809 Japanese Americans in California to test hypothesis of gradient differences based on country of residence. The most traditional Japanese Americans have a coronary heart disease as low as that observed in Japan. Those most acculturated to western culture have a three- to five-fold excess in coronary heart disease prevalence. Differences between these two groups are not accounted for by differences in the major risk factors of serum cholesterol, blood pressure, and smoking.

McGee, D., G. Rhoads, J. Hankin, K. Yano, and J. Tillotson. "Within-person variability of nutrient intake in a group of Hawaiian men of Japanese ancestry." AMER. J. CLIN. NUTR. 36 (1982): 657-663.

Seven day nutrient intake for 329 men in Hawaii finds that starch has small variance while polyunsaturated fatty acids have large variability. Except for these two nutrients and protein, there is very good agreement among nutrients in seven-day and 24-hour recall, the greater differences being between weekdays and weekends, the latter have higher intakes.

Miller, C.D. JAPANESE FOODS COMMONLY USED IN HAWAII. Honolulu, HI: University of Hawaii, 1933.

Although half a century old, this bulletin (Number 68) does an excellent job of explaining scientifically and in a practical manner many unusual Japanese ingredients including edamame, tofu, kirazu, tonyu, aburage, miso, natto, koji, konnyaku, umeboshi, hukusai, MSG, katsuo-bushi, iriko, the various seaweeds, noodles, fish and gluten cakes, kampyo, and goma that are so frequently consumed by the Japanese. Their nutrient content is discussed in a general way.

Miller, H.S., and S. Santo. "Nutritional improvement in Hokkaido orphanage children 1960-1970." J. AMER. DIETET. ASSOC. 72 (1978): 506-509.

More than 1400 children studied show growth improvement with diets that include milk and eggs. Consumption of additional foods show increase of stature and small weight differences.

Minowa, M., S. Bingham, and H.J. Cummings. "Dietary fibre intake in Japan." HUMAN NUTR: APPL. NUTR. 37A (1983): 113-119.

Total intake per capita in 1979 is 19.4 grams, with 5.1 grams coming from rice. Intakes in the ten largest cities are lower. Intakes are similar to those in Great Britain; therefore, fiber intakes cannot account for large bowel cancer rates in the two countries.

Nomura, A., B.E. Henderson, and J. Lee. "Breast cancer and diet among the Japanese in Hawaii." AMER. J. CLIN. NUTR. 31 (1978): 2020-2025.

The study investigates the diets of 86 male spouses of women with breast cancer. Their diets are higher in beef, meat, butter, margarine, cheese, corn, and weiners than are the diets of almost seven thousand other males whose wives did not develop the disease. The authors propose that if their diets are similar to those of their wives, this factor needs investigation.

Ohi, G., K. Minowa, T. Oyama, M. Nagahashi, N. Yamazaki, S. Yamamoto, K. Nagasako, K. Hayakaw, K. Kimura, and B. Mori. "Changes in dietary fiber intake among Japanese in the 20th century: A relationship to the prevalence of diverticular disease." AMER. J. CLIN. NUT. 38 (1983): 115-121.

The relationship between fiber intake and diverticular disease suggests threshold levels of fiber intake for the effective prevention of diverticular disease. Incidence is higher in the United States due to lower fiber intake.

Oiso, T. "Incidence of stomach cancer and its relation to dietary habits and nutrition in Japan between 1900 and 1975." CANCER RES. 35 (1975): 3254-3258.

Heavy rice and many salty foods are characteristics of the traditional Japanese diet; these and other factors are investigated in the country with the highest incidence of stomach cancer in the world. Forty percent of their calories come from boiled white rice, it may be 50 to 60% of the food consumed. Salty foods such as soybean paste, pickles, small fish or shellfish cooked with soy sauce, and seaweed are side dishes to complement the rice. Sake and sweet meats are made from rice. In some districts salt consumption is greater than 30 grams per day. Fat and oil content, although lower than in western countries is increasing in the diet as is animal protein. The author believes the continued high rate of stomach cancer is related to these dietary habits.

Sasaki, N. "Relationship of salt intake to hypertension in the Japanese diet." GERIATRICS. 10 (1964): 735-744.

Blood pressures in life insurance applicants the same in Japan as in the United States, but Japanese regional differences marked. Correlation exists between salt intake and mortality from apoplexy. National studies show intake primarily from soy sauce, table salt, miso, pickles, seasonings, salted fish, and preserved foods. Other considerations include the high intake of potassium and needed balance between sodium and potassium.

Ueshima, H., M. Kitada., M. Iida, M. Tanigaki, T. Shimamoto, M. Konishi, E. Nagano, N. Nakanishi, Y. Takamaya, H. Ozawa, and Y. Komachi. "Serum total cholesterol, triglyceride level, and dietary intake in Japanese students aged 15 years." AMER. J. EPIDEM. 116 (1982): 343-352.

The survey of 238 males and 217 females reveals serum cholesterol and triglyceride levels of 163.3mg/dl and 81.7mg/dl, respectively, for males, and 182.2mg/dl and 78.9mg/dl for females. Those females who participate in sports for three years have levels of cholesterol 10mg/dl lower than non-participants. Dietary intake of fat is 25-30% of energy and carbohydrate intake 55-61%.

Watanabe, T. M. Miyasaka, A. Koizumi, and M. Ikeda. "Regional difference in sodium chloride content in home-made and store-bought preparations of miso paste." TOHOKU J. EXPER. MED. 137 (1982): 305-311.

Miso, a fermentation product of salted soybeans and rice or soybeans and barley, is a leading source of sodium chloride in the diet. Homemade varieties varied from 9.1% to 18.2% while store-bought samples ranged from 10 to 12%. Correlations between areas and death rate indexes for cerebrovascular diseases are related to sodium chloride intake.

Wojtan, L.S. "Japanese food: A mirror of history." E. ASIAN OUTREACH INDIANA U. (Winter 1982-83): D1-2.

Discusses food preparation, changes in dietary pattern, rural and urban differences, and increase in popularity of Japanese foods in America. Lists the ten most popular Japanese foods in the United States, with tempura, chicken and beef teriyaki the top three. Ninety percent think Japanese food nutritious and nonfattening.

Yano, K., G.G. Rhoads, and A. Kagan. "Coffee, alcohol, and risk of coronary heart disease among Japanese men living in Hawaii." N. Eng. J. MED. 297 (1977): 405-409.

There is positive correlation between coffee intake and risk of coronary heart disease but it becomes statistically insignificant when cigarette smoking is taken into account.

Yoshioka, Y. FOOD AND AGRICULTURE IN JAPAN. Tokyo, Japan: Foreign Press Center, 1982.

Historical introduction and chapters on agricultural topics, food consumption, and nutrition. Includes calorie intake, dietary pattern information, per capita consumption data, and family food expenditures.

5.3   Resources for Recipes

Andoh, E. AN AMERICAN TASTE OF JAPAN. New York: William Morrow and Co., 1985.

Blends American and Japanese cuisines in the recipes after detailed introduction about buying and storing foodstuffs and equipment, detailed glossary as well.

Condon, C., and S. Ashiza. THE JAPANESE GUIDE TO FISH COOKING. Tokyo, Japan: Shufonotomo, 1978

Background information is given for 20 fish, including familiar, Japanese, and ideographic names, general materials, marketing and cooking suggestions, and two recipes. Fish terminology, folklore and general information precedes the glossary and the bilingual list of fish and fish products.

Doi, M. JAPANESE ONE-POT COOKERY. Tokyo, Japan: Kodansha International, 1966.

This award-winning volume, one of several by this author, has general background materials, types of nabe or casserole pots, recipes for fish, meat, and vegetable nabes, with pictures of each, spice and dip recipes, and a short glossary.

Egami, T. TYPICAL JAPANESE COOKING. Tokyo, Japan: Shibata Publishing Co., 1971.

Book is one of many by this radio and television cooking teacher. Background materials look at the country and culture and precede the recipes of common foods. Many color photographs show completed dishes.

Griffin, S. JAPANESE FOOD AND COOKING. Rutland, VT: Charles E. Tuttle Co., 1956.

More than 100 recipes in food category chapters precede one on festival dishes, table utensils, and table manners.

Hirasuna, D., and D.J. Hirasuna. FLAVORS OF JAPAN. San Francisco, CA: 101 Productions, 1981.

Collection of 175 classic and contemporary recipes, some typical only of home cooking, follow background food and culture information.

Keys, J.D. JAPANESE CUISINE, A CULINARY TOUR. Rutland, VT: Charles E. Tuttle Co., Inc., 1966.

Recipes are arranged by regions in Japan. There is a section on modern Tokyo cuisine and a very detailed glossary.

Kobayashi, K. SHOJIN COOKING, THE BUDDHIST VEGETARIAN COOK-BOOK. San Francisco, CA: The Buddhist Bookstore, 1977.

A short introduction is followed by the recipes, most of which originated in a monasterial lifestyle, and all follow traditional Buddhist precepts. The recipes are presented both by cooking technique and by food category groupings.

Kohno, S. HOME STYLE JAPANESE COOKING IN PICTURES. Tokyo, Japan: Shufunotomo Co., 1977.

Recipes, many with pictures of steps in the preparation, all with photographs of the finished product, are presented along with some arranged in typical or party menu item order.

Konishi, K. JAPANESE COOKING FOR HEALTH AND FITNESS. Woodbury, NY: Barron's Educational Series, 1984.

Each recipe has color photograph, many have step-by-step preparation photographs along with calorie, protein, fat, and carbohydrate content listings. The book features some sample menus based on consumption of 1600 calories a day. Party menus are given with suggestions for order of preparation and serving.

Kushi, A.T. HOW TO COOK WITH MISO. Tokyo, Japan: Japan Publications, 1978.

Text includes yin/yang and other health considerations, how to use miso, and how to make it. A glossary of foods and equipment, tables of composition of soybean products, barleys, rice, and miso are included.

Ma, N.C., S. Ma, and H.M. Yamawaki. MRS. MA'S JAPANESE COOKING. Tokyo, Japan: Japan Publications, 1980.

Recipes are presented in food category chapters with photographs of the step-by-step preparations and the completed dish.

Martin, J., and P. Martin. JAPANESE COOKING. New York: Signet Books, 1970.

More than 200 recipes follow introductory section on the cuisine and dining. Each food category chapter begins with considerable cultural and informative material. Glossary of ingredients and equipment.

Omae, K., and Y. Tachibana. THE BOOK OF SUSHI. Tokyo, Japan: Kodansha International, 1981.

How to order and eat at a sushi bar or shop, including vocabulary, start this beautifully photographed volume. The main sushi fish are discussed and shown. List of equipment and preparation instructions are followed by a description of a fish market; other chapters include sushi design, its history, and nutrition.

Ortiz, E.L., with M. Endo. THE COMPLETE BOOK OF JAPANESE COOKING. New York: M. Evans and Co., 1976.

Introductory materials include many line drawings of equipment and ingredients. Recipes are in food category chapters with many master recipes and variations for them. Seven New Year recipes, typical menus, and a glossary are included.

Shurtleff, W., and A. Aoyagi. THE BOOK OF TOFU. Brookline, MA: Autumn Press, 1975.

Has more than 500 recipes for this soybean product, along with history and practical information such as how to make it. Describes soybean as milk and in every form imaginable. The traditional tofu shop and modern tofu making are two of its chapters. Also contains sources of solidifiers, shops, and bibliography. Other books by this husband and wife team include THE BOOK OF MISO, THE BOOK OF TEMPEH, and THE BOOK OF KUDZU, each treating these foods in the same thorough manner.

Slack, S.F. JAPANESE COOKING. Tuscon, AZ: HP Books, 1985.

Some background material, an extensive glossary of ingredients, equipment, including knives, and a chapter on garnishes precede the recipes. Many color photographs in this paperback.

Tokimasa, E.C. JAPANESE FOODS. Honolulu, HI: Temmy, 1982.

This revised and expanded volume of more than 300 recipes (originally published by the Hui Foundation, in 1951, 1956, and 1969) has easy to follow recipes presented in food category chapters.

Tsuji, S. JAPANESE COOKING, A SIMPLE ART. Tokyo, Japan: Kodansha International, 1980.

Details cooking concepts, food lore, and recipes and discusses the essence as
well as the details of Japanese cooking. After an introduction, the 20 chapters
are lessons in basic Japanese cooking methods. This section with about 90
recipes is followed by 130 selected recipes, some simple, others advanced.

Chapter 6

OTHER ASIAN AMERICANS

6.1 Introduction

The influx of Southeast Asian refugees into the United States represents a unique challenge for them and for those who come in contact with them. Assimilation into American society has been and continues to be part of the strength of this country. The greatest number of new immigrants come from the Caribbean, South America, and Southeast Asia. The first two groups have an advantage of the same alphabet; as English-speaking natives those from southeast Asia have to learn alphabet, language, and a culture far different from anything they have known before. This has not stopped the waves of Asian immigrants but it does present a formidable challenge to them and to those in health care, community related facilities, and to us, their neighbors.

Limited information has been published about the everyday foods of other peoples from this part of the world. Little is known of their food preferences, their customs, and/or their nutritional status. Much of what is known about their foods represents what they believe westerners want to know, what they eat on holidays or special occasions, or what very affluent people from their lands report they eat. Furthermore, peoples from this part of the world have very much the same problems as do Blacks or Hispanics, they are viewed as one group, considered in the aggregate and not seen as individual people from individual countries, from local regions, or from special groups within either of these.

What follows is a short synopsis and introduction. It is an appetizer to whet the appetite for additional knowledge. The Southeast Asian groups listed are those with the largest numbers immigrating to the United States. Other groups have arrived in smaller numbers and are omitted from this listing.

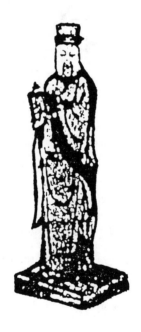

6.2   Korean Americans

Korean food habits are very much like those of the Chinese, coupled with considerable Japanese influence. They cook in woks, cut most of their food into small pieces, use chopsticks, and serve their food all at once, not in courses.

All meals begin with a very, very spicy pickled vegetable dish called "kimchee". Usually it is made of cabbage seasoned with hot peppers, but it can be made with other vegetables. Meat and seafood are eaten in abundance as are vegetables. Many of the meats are barbecued. Korean food is hearty and boldly flavored.

Meals include rice served alone or mixed with other grains, vegetables, meats, and mixed meat and fish dishes. Milk and milk products are not part of the Korean meal pattern. Neither are desserts, though these are always served when guests come to dinner or on other festive occasions.

The Koreans use more meat than do either the Chinese or the Japanese; because of this, fat consumption is high. If given a choice of meats, beef is most often selected. Sesame oil is preferred for cooking, not the corn, peanut, or soybean oils the Chinese use. The beverage of choice is not tea. It may be soup, or it may be hot water poured into the charred rice or barley pot. It may also be a soybean paste liquid or a ginseng drink.

In the country breakfast is the main meal of the day, in the city it is supper. Rice is preferred at breakfast, noodles are popular for lunch, and rice and/or another grain is served at dinner. Rice, soup, and kimchee are by far the most popular foods at mealtimes. Many of the dishes can be very spicy as chili sauces and hot peppers are favorites in this cuisine. These spicy foods are less popular at snack times, instead steamed rice cookies, dried fruits, seeds, and nuts are eaten. Garlic, green onions, sesame seeds, chili peppers, ginger, soy sauce, and vinegar flavor most meals along with the kimchee. Vegetables are liked but often only eaten fresh in summer; they are eaten pickled year round.

Health problems have been reported in this population, many related to poor diet prior to immigration. Others are related to excessive use of salt and the consumption of large quantities of pickled vegetable products.

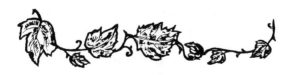

6.3   Cambodian Americans

The people from Cambodia do not eat their food with chopsticks or use rice bowls. They use plates, forks, and spoons. Knife use at the table is still considered barbaric and knives do not appear at the table in Cambodia.

Food tastes and looks Chinese but with some differences. Here noodles are a breakfast food and rice, still the main grain as it is for those of southern China, is served at lunch and dinner. Tea consumption is low, warm and hot water are beverages of choice at meals, and between meals, too.

All meats but mutton are popular, fish is used a great deal, and poultry is not too popular. The fish sauces used have peanuts added. Like the Vietnamese, Cambodians like raw vegetables and salads. They are served with very pungent sauces. Meal patterns for the main meals are like those of the Chinese. Snack patterns differ, Cambodians consume many, many snacks, while the Chinese consume few, if any.

6.4   Laotian Americans

The food habits of the people from Laos are very much like those of their Cambodian neighbors, with seasonings added. These include lemon grass and coriander, items included in almost every dish.

Forks and spoons are the utensils of choice; fingers are used, too. Most of the dishes of this cuisine mix many ingredients together. The Laotians are are fond of the banana, it is used frequently and in many ways. They use its leaves to wrap foods and the fruit is enjoyed fried or fresh. Other fruits are popular; they are eaten raw.

Curries are used in Laos; these are more popular than are seasonings derived from chili peppers alone. Rice is the main grain, preferred as sticky or glutinous rice. It is a very short and fat grain of rice. The Laotians eat it in quantity at the table and in their sweet dishes. Other Asian populations prefer sweet rice only in sweet items and stuffings. For Laotians, rice is served at all meals and sometimes combined with black beans or yams.

Another item of difference between Laotian foods and those of other countries in this region of the world is that many Laotian dishes require long cooking and they rely on fresh rather than preserved or pickled ingredients. With these long cooked items, the people of Laos like tea or coffee, more often the latter, and serve it black or with sugar and cream.

6.5   Thai American

Cooking of Thailand, the country that was once known as Siam, is rich and varied and has many unusual flavors. The principal culinary influence is Chinese and foods are stir fried, steamed, or grilled, preferable over charcoal. There is also some Indian influence seen in Thai curries, stewed dishes, and sweets. These sweets are popular as snack foods and are consumed frequently. Use of fish, coconut milk, lemon grass, chili peppers, coriander, fish sauce, garlic, herbs, and spices abound. Of all the countries in this region, the foods of this cuisine are often the hottest.

Rice is the staple grain and "kaengs" or curries and fried or steamed food accompany it. It is consumed in very large quantities; to eat at least a pound a day is quite common. Soups are popular. Dinners often have two desserts if there are guests, none if just the family is present. To eat these dinners, forks are used to push food onto large spoons which are carried to the mouth. Beverages served at meals vary. They may be tea and/or fruit drinks.

Breakfast includes a bowl of rice soup with many spicy seasoning items. Large quantities of food are not typical, people from Thailand prefer to eat a little at a time, but many times during the day. Noodles in soup for lunch; if not served, are stir fried with combinations of meats and vegetables. The main meal of the day is in the evening. It is composed of many foods brought to the table as soon as they are cooked and in no particular order. Salads and/or yams are used between hot dishes to cool the palate; it is not uncommon to have several at the dinner meal along with several other dishes, none consumed in large amounts. If dessert is served for the family, it is generally simple; the preference is for fresh fruits.

6.6   Malaysian American

Cooking of Malaysia is mentioned here because it bears resemblance to many of those just mentioned as well as a few others and because some Asian immigrants have lived there for some time. Malaysian cooking is a blend or marriage of Chinese, Indian, Cambodian, Laotian, Thai, and Malay influences. However, one major difference is that many Malays are Moslems, so pork and alcoholic beverages are forbidden.

Rice is served at all meals and dishes that accompany it are rich and spicy. They are flavored with ginger, chili peppers, and often prawns. Malaysians love sweet desserts, as do the Cambodians, and for them and the people from Thailand, tea and fruit beverages are popular. They also like coffee.

Traditionally eating was done with the fingers, nowadays spoons and forks are very popular. In Singapore, foods of many cuisines such as Malay, Japanese, and Indian are eaten alone or in combination at any meal of the day, but particularly at main meals. Peculiar to Singapore is Nonya or Peranakan food. This style of food is a mixture of Chinese ingredients and Malay spices.

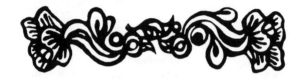

6.7   Vietnamese Americans

The food habits of Vietnamese who have come to the United States are similar to Chinese immigrants from Sichuan and Hunan. Similarities exist in terms of basic preparation and use of ingredients. The spicing makes them subtly different and the soy sauce used changes their flavor, too.

The Vietnamese soy sauce is called "nuoc nam" and is a fish soy with a strong fishy odor but a very mild taste. It is the basic ingredient in many Vietnamese dishes and gives them a characteristic taste. Spicing differences are regional, black pepper and ginger are used frequently in the north, chili peppers are in greater use in the south.

There is a French influence in this cuisine, at the table and in the diet; it can most easily be seen as French bread is served with the Chinese style meals and eaten with chopsticks. The French influence is also noticeable in the use of pates, often made with fish. There are some lesser Indian influences, too. These include use of curries with potatoes and asparagus.

Unlike the Chinese, the Vietnamese eat a good many salads. They prefer chicken over pork, both cooked with very little fat. All foods are eaten with polished long grain rice, the staple of the diet. Rice noodles are also popular. Eggs are liked very much and often indulged in quite heavily. Tropical fruits are preferred, as are tropical vegetables.

Fish and seafood are popular. They are eaten not only fresh but in fish pastes, and in the pate form. Many of these are heavily salted. Like Koreans and southwestern Chinese from the Sichuan and Hunam provinces, chili peppers and chili pastes are used frequently, along with vinegars. There is also a penchant for lemons and limes, a predominant flavor in many dishes.

Vietnamese share the oriental dislike for milk and milk products, consume a lot of fruits and vegetables both plain and mixed with meat dishes, and eat many sweets in small cakes, candies, and sweetened beverages. Milk, if drunk, is often one or two tablespoons of condensed milk stirred into a glass of water.

Breakfast is more western because of their consumption of bread or croissant and because they like coffee with sugar and some cream. These accompany soup with rice or noodles and meat. Tea is the beverage of choice at lunch and dinner. The preferred cooking fat at breakfast, lunch, or dinner is often lard; when that is not available or affordable, vegetable oils are used. For croissants, however, butter is used as do the French.

6.8   Overall

Several common health problems among peoples from Southeast Asia include intestinal parasites, skin infections, and dental caries. These and generalized undernutrition often result from problems prior to immigration. Iron deficiency anemias, low calcium intakes, and poor growth rates have been reported in the United States.

The best way to learn about these peoples is to read articles, books, and cookbooks about them. In the books and articles are cultural information items and health related materials. In the cookbooks is a wealth of information about meal preparation, planning, ingredients, and related items of culture.

Their food habits like their health problems exhibit more similarities to each other than they do those of the western world.

While there are similarities in foods and in preparation techniques, there are also differences. Because of these differences, and the differences of language and culture, reading is not enough. Experience the tastes by trying to cook them at home, frequenting ethnic restaurants if nearby, and exchanging information with people of the ethnic groups or with those who know peoples of these cultures.

Consult the reference and resource listings for reading materials and the local telephone directories for locations of eateries and associations.

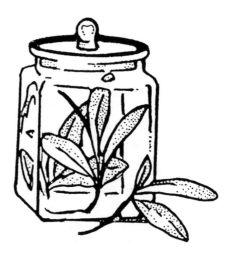

6.9   Asian References

6.9.1   Korean

Chai, R.S., O.K. Ahn, and M.J. Kim. "Amino acid content of Korean food." Vth INTER. CONG NUTR. September (1960): 53.

Many foods, including fermented ones and seaweed, and the overall Korean diet are analyzed for ten amino acids.

Kang, T.S., and G.E. Kang. "Adjustment patterns of Korean-American elderly: Case studies of ideal types." J. MINOR. AGING 8 (1983): 47-55.

Uses modified typology of anomie theory to examine five basic types of adaptive behavior among recently arrived Korean elderly.

Kim, K.K., M.B. Kohrs, and M.R. Grier. "Dietary intakes of elderly Korean Americans." J. AMER. DIETET. ASSOC. 2 (1984): 164-169.

Study of 40 elderly Koreans, using 24-hour dietary recall, shows mean intake of the men at 92% of RDA while intake of the women is only 60% RDA. Men meet their RDA's for phosphorus and protein while up to 16% of the women have less than 66% RDA for these nutrients. Milk and ice cream are the major calcium rich foods consumed but only 23% of this population actually consumes more than one cup of them per day.

Lee, H.O., and S.H. Kim. "A study on every possible correlation between daily food intake and growth rate of senior high school students." KOR. J. NUTR 6,3 (1973): 197-206.

One hundred boys and girls doing seven-day recalls indicate they had been breast fed. Their calorie and vitamins A and C and thiamin intake are below recommended levels with 73% of calories from carbohydrates, 14% from protein, and 13% from fat for the boys, 65, 14, and 21%, respectively for girls. Calorie and physical growth correlation is significant at the .05 level as it is for protein intake. Favorite snacks are fruits, juice, milk, and ice cream.

Lien, N.M., K.K. Meyer, and M. Winick. "Early malnutrition and late adoption: A study of their effects on the development of Korean orphans adopted into American families." AMER. J. CLIN. NUTR. 30 (1977): 1734-1739.

Studies 240 orphans adopted after age two and finds that though they surpass Korean natives, they never catch up to American reference standards for height, weight, and academic performance if they were severely malnourished before adoption. Moderately and well nourished children score above the average in school suggesting that attainment may reflect stimulatory effect of their new home.

Park, C.S. "Studies on the mineral contents in Korean foods." KOR. J. NUTR. 7 (1974): 31-36.

Sodium and potassium content in Korean fruits and vegetables are reported. Unusual items include leaves and stems given separately in green leafy vegetables, whole, skin, and pulp given for what they refer to as fruit vegetables (eggplants, tomatoes, cucumbers, onions, peppers, and burdock) and whole, skin, and pulp of fruits.

6.9.2 Laotian

Holton, N.R. "Health care problems among Southeast Asian refugees." MINN. MED. 62 (1979): 633-634.

Identifies health needs of more than 1,500 Hmong from Laos who have settled in St. Paul, Minnesota. Incidence of tuberculosis, parasitic infections, upper respiratory infections among children, gout, nutritional problems, and cultural problems such as eschewing cold foods during the first post-partum month are problems encountered.

INTRODUCTION TO VARIOUS ETHNIC GROUPS FROM LAOS. New York: Lutheran Immigration and Refugee Service of the Lutheran Council of New York, 1982.

Details Tai, Mon, Khmer, Hmong, and Yao groups and lists other available materials about these ethnic groups in this six-page reprint.

Olness, K. "Cultural aspects in working with Lao refugees." MINN. MED. 62, (1979): 871-874.

Case study serves as introduction to culture, calendar, ceremonies, life cycle events, codes of behavior, and typical foods and medicines. Taboos, such as knife use in crib slats in the hospital, prohibition against eating in a reclining position, and others are detailed.

6.9.3   Thai

Keusch, G.T., F.J. Troncale, L.H. Miller, V. Promadhat, and P.R. Anderson.
"Acquired lactose malabsorption in Thai children." PEDIAT. 43 (1969):
540-545.

Studies 172 Thai infants and children and finds lactose tolerance flat in 14%
of the infants under one year of age, and in 87% of those over two years showing
increase of intolerance as they age. By age five, 85% are intolerant or have
lactose maldigestion.

Potter, S.H. FAMILY LIFE IN A NORTHERN THAI VILLAGE. Berkeley,
CA: University of California Press, 1977.

Chapter on economic life includes foods typical to the Thai diet and the roles
family members play in its preparation. Rest of the volume gives a clear picture
of the family system and its importance in this culture group.

Schumaker, J.F. "Eating patterns in Thailand." OBESITY BARIATRIC
MED. 12,3 (1983): 71-73.

Investigates attitudes toward and eating patterns related to obesity in 221
middle class Thais. only seven percent are found to be obese yet 72% say they
overeat. In addition, 89% indicate they they sometimes eat when they do not
feel hungry. Reasons for this, their rare participation in any type of exercise,
and lack of obesity are explored.

Visudhiphan, S. Poolsuppasit, O. Piboonnukarintr, and S. Tumliang. "The
relationship between high fibrinolytic activity and daily capsicum ingestion in Thais." AMER. J. CLIN. NUTR. 35 (1982): 1452-1458.

Study shows that capsicum, a hot seasoning agent used daily in Thai cuisine, is found to induce increased fibrinolytic activity and simultaneously causes
hypocoagulability. Fibrinolytic activity is significantly higher in 88 Thais, not
in 55 Americans residing in Thailand, and the Thais have higher antithrombin
II.

6.9.4   Vietnamese

Anh, N.T., T.K. Thuc, and J.D. Welsh. "Lactose malabsorption in adult
Vietnamese." AMER. J. CLIN. NUTR. 30 (1977): 468-469.

Lactose malabsorption tested in 31 Vietnamese adults shows all had malabsorption, 20 having symptoms during and after the tests. Diet histories reveal 23 consumed one to three glasses of milk a day in Vietnam and eight noticed the symptoms there. In the United States, 30 drink milk and six have symptoms. Group has 174 siblings and all consume milk; in Vietnam it was canned, usually sweetened, or powdered, and only occasionally fresh.

Brink, M.S., P. Page, N. Truitner, and L.S. Nelson. GETTING TO KNOW THE VIETNAMESE FOOD HABITS AND CULTURE. St. Paul, MN: University of Minnesota, Cooperative Extension, 1976.

Eight-page booklet about food habits, food preparation, and foods used in the Vietnamese diet. The Vietnamese foods given are grouped in the four food groups.

Carlson, E., M. Kipps, and J. Thomson. "Feeding the Vietnamese in the United Kingdom and the rationale behind their food habits." PROC. NUTR. SOC. 41 (1982): 229-237.

Interviews with incoming Vietnamese refugees reveal diets high in carbohydrates and low in fat. It is close to recommendations and should be copied by nationals, not have them adapt to UK diets.

Carlson, E., M. Kipps, and J. Thompson. "Feeding Vietnamese refugees in the United Kingdom." J. AMER. DIETET. ASSOC. 81 (1982): 164-167.

Study shows that each meal in each day is equally important and that it revolves around the family. Rice is the staple of the diet and the single most important food, providing 40% of their energy and 20% of the day's protein. Dairy products are rarely consumed, more calcium and vitamin D intake is needed, and consumption of fruits and vegetables, high in Vietnam, is reduced in the United States because of cost.

Casey, P., and I. Harrill. "Nutrient intake of Vietnamese women relocated in Colorado." NUTR. REP. INTERNATIONAL 16 (1977): 687-693.

Data from 24-hour recalls of 30 Vietnamese women show prevalence of traditional food patterns with American foods supplementing them. With exception of iron, calcium, and zinc, the mean intakes meet the RDAs. Older women, ages 51-65, do not meet RDAs except for protein and vitamin C. Tables show intake of all nutrients by age groups, education, and number of different foods consumed.

Crane, N.T., and N.R. Green. "Food habits and food preferences of Vietnamese refugees living in northern Florida." J. AMER. DIETET. ASSOC. 76 (1980): 591-593.

Changes in food habits, frequency of consumption and food related problems associated with relocation are studied in a mail-in questionnaire. Thirty percent were returned indicating rice, fresh vegetables, milk, soft drinks, and cooking oil are consumed the most, five to six times per week with milk and soft drinks significantly increased from use in Vietnam. Fish and tea consumption is down since immigration. Steak is the only food listed that is liked more than Vietnamese foods.

Crawford, A.C. CUSTOMS AND CULTURE OF VIETNAM. Rutland, VT: Charles E. Tuttle Co., 1966.

Chapters on the country, people, religion, education and communication, health and welfare, and other topics offer good introductory information. Valuable for general background even though it refers specifically to time when American military were in Vietnam.

Dobbins, E., D.K. Fischer, and M.C.S. Santopietro. "A beginner's guide to Vietnamese culture." REG. NURSE (January 1981): n.p.

Discusses individual, family, and community health concepts in terms of religion, self, and cultural factors.

Eichelberger, B.J., and L.W. Miller. "Dietary habits and nutritional problems of Vietnamese refugees." W.I.C. NOTES 4 (1981): four unnumbered pages.

Common health problems are large number of positive reactions for tuberculosis tests, high incidence of intestinal parasites, scabies, fungal infections, dental caries, and generalized undernutrition. Dietary beliefs, practices related to health, consumer behavior, meal patterns, adequacy of the diet, common nutrition problems generalized.

Holtzman, M., N. Azuaje, R. Rodriguez, and A. Laverty. TET CELEBRATING THE VIETNAMESE NEW YEAR. Westminster, CA: Westminster School District Staff, 1981.

Details the three day holiday of Tet; includes calendar, preparations, dressing, foods, games, poetry, music, theater, and art, all important parts of this important holiday. Only one recipe given in the hundred plus pages of thorough view of items of importance to this culture.

Hong, N.K. VIETNAMESE THEMES. New York: Board of Education of the City of New York, 1981.

Lists cultural differences between Americans and Vietnamese, with matching columns regarding affections, habits, holidays, cooking and eating, housing, and much more. Bibliography included.

Manderson, L., and M. Mathews. "Vietnamese attitudes towards maternal and infant health." MED. J. AUSTRALIA 1 (1981): 69-72.

Humoral classifications show only minor modification with migration to Australia for Vietnamese pregnant women. Traditional practices of infant feeding are changing with short period of breast feeding or exclusive use of bottle and the early introduction of solid foods.

Manderson, L., and M. Mathews. "Vietnamese behavioral and dietary precautions during pregnancy." ECOL. FD. NUTR. 11,1 (1981): 1-8.

Important cultural restrictions for 40 ethnic Vietnamese and Vietnamese Chinese women include need for women to remain active, not eat culturally described hot foods during the first trimester, eat specially considered tonic foods, and eat culturally considered cold foods in the second trimester, and eat even more of them in the third trimester. Other foods are pro or prescribed and are listed in tables. Other Asian cultures differ with respect to these concerns of pregnancy and are discussed.

Mathews, M., and L. Manderson. "Infant feeding practices and lactation diets amongst Vietnamese immigrants." AUST. PAEDIATRIC J. 16 (1980): 263-266.

Interviews with 40 women showed that humoral pathology of hot and cold food classifications affected their diets and those of their infants. Declines in incidence and duration of breast feeding, earlier introduction of solid foods, and increased use of commercially manufactured baby foods were practiced primarily by women with babies born in Australia.

Stephenson, S. "The feeding of Vietnamese children." FD. MGT. 14,8 (1979): 32-36.

Experience of school food service director as 60 Vietnamese arrive on their first day in school is the setting of article detailing the food culture of the students and their families and the culture in general.

Thuy, T.N., H.D. Tam, W.J. Craig, and G. Zimmerman. "Food habits and preferences of Vietnamese children." J. SCH. HEALTH 53,2 (1983): 144-147.

Questionnaire explores food habits of 70 children, comparing food habits of recent and earlier arrivals. Older children consumed peanut butter, ice cream, pies, and milkshakes more frequently than did similar age new arrivals. Other differences are found in younger children. The majority of children of all ages eat fruits as snacks. Use of rice, eggs, cheese, milk, meats, and fruit juice is not significantly different regardless of age.

Waldman, E.B., S.B. Lege, B. Oseid, and J.P. Carter. "Health and nutritional status of Vietnamese refugees." SOUTH. MED. J. 72 (1979): 1300-1303.

Paper summarizes health and nutritional information on Vietnamese refugees in the United States. Main problems include dental caries, tuberculosis, skin infestations, inadequate immunizations, and limited access to health care.

6.9.5 Mixed Southeast Asian

Please note: These items address one or more groups and/or they relate to the countries above, or to others in Asia.

Abraham, R. "Trace element intake by Asians during pregnancy." PROC. NUTR. SOC. 41 (1982): 261-265.

Study uses seven-day dietary recall and shows that copper levels in vegetarians and non-vegetarian Asians are low. Zinc intakes are lower in the vegetarian Asians than in the non-vegetarians, and they have high phytate/zinc ratios.

ASIAN FOODS GUIDE FOR TEACHERS. Sacramento CA: The Dairy Council of California, n.d.

Booklet done with help of several other agencies discusses Korean, Chinese, Japanese, Vietnamese, Cambodian, Laotian, and Thai food practices in terms of typical meal patterns and foods eaten from the basic four food groups. A glossary of typical foods from each group has phonetic translations. In Chinese, they are in both Cantonese and Mandarin.

Backas, N. "Exotic Asian cuisine spices American menus." REST. INST. 94 (1984): 163+.

Discusses ethnic differences between Koreans and Thai, including Korean preference for beef, grilling, and liberal use of spices compared to heavy use of spices, curries, basil, and coriander by people from Thailand. Glossary of ingredients and some recipes given.

Borchardt, K.A., H. Ortega, J.D. Mahood, J. Newman, P.R. DeLay, J. Doss, K. Hopkins, G. Schecter, and R.H. Gelber. "Intestinal parasites in Southeast Asian refugees." WEST. J. MED. 135 (1981): 93-96.

Surveys 6,241 Southeast Asian refugees, countries of origin not given, and indicates that 32.9% harbor one or more parasites, helmiths being the most frequent isolate.

Breitenbucher, R.B. "Medical care of Southeast Asians – Compliance." MINN. MED. 63 (1980): 41-44.

Article discusses dietary and medical compliance of Southeast Asians, who the author readily admits are not a single cultural entity.

Buchholz, M. "Special help for Southeast Asian refugees." FD. NUTR. 14 (1984): 4-7.

Special slide-tape sets on shopping in supermarkets available in six Southeast Asian languages and in English explaining checkout procedures, how to differentiate between food and non-food items, the importance of not opening packages to check contents, and other mysteries Asians need help with in the American market-place. Tips include ways to tailor nutrition education to the various backgrounds, adapt materials, and use teaching tools.

Bullard, B.M. ASIA IN NEW YORK CITY. New York: The Asia Society, 1981.

While much of the information is local – films, radio, television, societies, churches, businesses, libraries, educational institutions, consular offices, and the like – all are excellent sources for reference materials; addresses and phone numbers are included.

Campbell, M., and R. Loewen. "The food habits of Southeast Asian refugees – Implications in the Canadian setting." CAN. J. HOME ECON. 31,2 (1981): 92-95.

Overviews diet of Vietnamese, Laotian, and Cambodian refugees, looks at the basic food groups for use and avoidance. Suggestions are made to work with diets; valuable as introduction to the problems in general.

Cantazaro, A., and R.J. Moser. "Health status of Refugees from Vietnam, Laos, and Cambodia." J. AMER. MED. ASSOC. 247 (1982): 1303-1308.

Evaluates 709 refugees within two months of resettlement and found 61% have intestinal parasites, 55% positive tuberculin test results, 37% anemia, 14% hepatitus B, and 12% abnormal VDRL. Except for hepatitus, significant differences were noted among ethnic groups.

Chow, E. "Cultural health traditions: Asian perspectives." PROVIDING SAFE NURSING CARE FOR ETHNIC PEOPLE OF COLOR. Edited by M.F. Branch and P.P. Paxton. New York: Appleton Century Crofts, 1976, pp. 99-114.

While Asian is defined as Chinese, Japanese, Korean, and Filipino, the chapter focuses on the Chinese system of medicine with its emphasis on prevention. Comparisons to and analyses of the other Asian groups is in a short introductory section. Chinese medicine is discussed in detail.

Crouch, A.R., editor. MID-ATLANTIC DIRECTORY TO RESOURCES FOR ASIAN STUDIES. Washington, DC: Mid-Atlantic Region Association for Asian Studies, 1980.

Includes organizations, curriculum development and services, colleges, universities, and academic associations, libraries and information services, bookstores and publishers, museums, galleries, and places to visit. Most but not all entries limited to this region of the country.

CULTURAL TEACHING KIT # 2. Sacramento, CA: Department of Health Services, November 1981.

Resource materials include selected nutrition education pamphlets translated into Cambodian, Laotian, and Vietnamese, literature about the Asian cultures, and a selection of pamphlets centered on the theme of foods for women, infants, and children.

Curtis, S. "A taster's guide to three oriental cuisines." FOOD AND WINE (June 1983): 14-16.

Discusses Thai, Vietnamese, and Korean foods offering a brief introduction to each of them. Common dishes including beverages are described. Restaurants in seven cities are suggested.

Erickson, R.V., and G.N. Hoang. "Health problems among Indochinese refugees." AMER. J. PUBLIC HEALTH 70 (1980): 1003-1006.

The results of medical evaluations of 194 refugees indicate a significant number of hematological (37%), dermatological (26%), psychiatric (10% of adults), and thyroid (5%) abnormalities. Refugees are from Vietnam (61%), Laos (32%), and Cambodia (7%). Tuberculosis, intestinal parasitism, skin infections, malaria, HbSAg carrier state, anemia, hemoglobin disorders, dental caries, and poor dentition are prevalent.

"Exotic Far Eastern fare." SCH. FOODSER. J. 32,3 (1978): 45+.

Background information focuses on the popularity and cultural significance of rice, some customs, recipes, and geographical information.

Fujii, S.M. "Elderly Asian Americans and use of public services." SOCIAL CASEWK. (March 1976): 202-207.

Various studies reviewed show service utilization is low and not likely top increase although numbers increase and family traditions change.

Gee, E. COUNTERPOINT. Los Angeles, CA: Asian American Studies Center, University of California, 1975, pp. 563-586.

Asian American census highlights of 1970 include family characteristics, educational background, employment and income information, and sources of income for Chinese, Japanese, Pilipino (their spelling), Korean, and Hawaiian populations. Tables of other data, including immigration, and a bibliography compiled by C. Lee follow.

Glass, R.I., P. Nieburg, R. Cates, C. Davis, R. Russbach, S. Peel, H. Nothdurft, and R. Turnbull. "Rapid assessment of health status and preventive medicine needs of newly arrived Kampuchean refugees, Sa Kaeo, Thailand." LANCET (April 19, 1980): 868-872.

Simple epidemiological techniques reduce morbidity and mortality, particularly among children aged four who showed highest risk of death. Intervention techniques needed are for measles vaccination. Absence of vitamin deficiencies obviate the need for immediate supplementation. Malaria and tuberculosis are major problems.

Go, K. THE FOOD HABITS AND PRACTICES OF SOUTHEAST ASIANS, PRIMARILY CAMBODIANS AND LAOTIANS. Alameda, CA: County Health Care Services Agency, 1979.

Report aids professionals in providing nutritional guidance in assessing patterns, habits, and preferences. Gives information on the cultural food practices of the two groups, available services, and list of local Asian food sources.

Hallberg, L., E. Bjorn-Rasmissen, L. Rossander, and R. Suwanik. "Iron absorption from Southeast Asian diets." AMER. J. CLIN. NUTR. 30 (1977): 539-548.

Implicates two main factors in earlier studies, the homogenization of the labeled meals before serving and the use of rice flour instead of rice. Iron absorption is higher than previously reported, on average 0.16mg, and is consistent with the actual prevalence of iron deficiency. The article discusses a number of factors that can be used to facilitate design and interpretation of dietary iron absorption.

Hallberg, L., E. Bjorn-Rasmussen, L. Rossander, R. Suwanik, R. Pleehachinda, and M. Tuntawiroon. "Iron absorption from some Asian meals containing contamination iron." AMER. J. CLIN. NUTR. 37 (1983): 272-277.

The extent of isotopic exchange, the native iron, and the contamination iron (from the soil) is measured in vitro. Results imply it is essential to consider the presence of contamination iron and its limited bioavailability; up to 50% of the nonheme iron in the 12 Asian meals of 85 subjects did not exchange with the added inorganic radioiron tracer in the extrinsic tag method used.

Hankin, J.H., C.S. Chung, and M.K.W. Kau. "Genetic and epidemiologic studies of oral characteristics in Hawaii's schoolchildren: Dietary patterns and caries prevalence." J. DENTAL RES. 52 (1973): 1079-1086.

Shows relationship between candy and gum intake and caries in 910 students. There is a significant amount of ethnic variation with Hawaiian children doing best, Japanese second best, and Caucasians poorest. Bread and cereal eating are negatively associated, candy and gum are positively associated with caries in two 24-hour recalls of 39 food items.

Ho, G.P.A. "Factors affecting adaptation to American dietary pattern by students from the oriental countries." Ph.D. dissertation. Pennsylvania State University, 1961.

Analyzes students from India, China, Japan, Korea, Thailand, Indonesia, Ceylon, and Pakistan to compare what was and is eaten. Nationality and degree of adaptation were significant, with Indians having the highest adaptation and Chinese the lowest. There was no relationship between food adaptation and having tasted American food in their native countries.

Hollingsworth, A.O., L.P. Brown, and D.A. Brooten. "The refugees and childbearing: What to expect." REG. NURSE (November 1980): 45-48.

Case study serves as focus for discussion of why Vietnamese fathers rarely participate in the births of their children and of other concerns they and others in the region share. For instance, Cambodian women won't want to see outsiders for three days after birth, Vietmanese babies are dressed in old clothes, and shampooing after delivery is not acceptable behavior. Postpartum food preferences are important to this population, they should include rice, pork, chicken, and salty foods.

Hoang, G.N., and R.V. Erickson. "Guidelines for providing medical care to Southeast Asian refugees." J. AMER. MED. ASSOC. 248 (1982): 710-714.

Discusses historical and socioeconomic background cultural traits and beliefs, traditional concepts of health and disease, and recommends health services. Provides list of culturally offensive practices, as well.

Hundley, N., Jr., editor. THE ASIAN AMERICAN; THE HISTORICAL EXPERIENCE. Santa Barbara, CA: Clio Press, 1976.

Chinese, Japanese, Filipino, Korean, and East Indian communities are explored in terms of ideas and ways of life. While the approach is historical in nature, it helps gain insights into the behaviors of these ethnic groups.

Intengan, C.L. "Nutritional evaluation of breast-feeding practices in some countries in the Far East." J. TROP. PED. ENVIR. CHILD HEALTH 2 (1976): 63-67.

Discusses breast feeding in Taiwan, Indonesia, Japan, Hong Kong, Philippines, and China, as reported in 17 research reports. Points out differences in duration, addition of other foods, and urban and rural areas. Gives reasons for weaning, milk substitutes, and food supplements.

James, C., and D. McCaskill. "Rice in the American diet." CER. FDS. WORLD 28 (1983): 667-669.

Stresses usage in American market.

Johnson, L.D., and L.A. Wilson. "Influence of soybean variety and the method of processing in tofu manufacturing: Comparison of methods for measuring soluble solids in soymilk." J. FOOD SCI. 49 (1984): 202-204.

Explains the two main processes for making tofu or beancurd from three different varieties of soybean and determines accuracy in several methods of determining percent solids.

Johnson, R.C., R.E. Cole, F.M. Ahern, S.Y. Schwitters, E.H. Ahern, Y.H.
   Huang, R.M. Johnson, and J.Y. Park. "Reported lactose tolerance of
   various racial/ethnic groups in Hawaii and Asia." BEHAV. GEN. 10
   (1980): 377-385.

Intolerance symptoms are infrequent among various racial/ethnic groups in
Hawaii and homeland Chinese, Japanese, and Koreans in this self reporting
study of milk consumed in childhood and adulthood. Study supports of the
belief that dietary practices influence tolerance, these are substantiated in the
more than 1,200 subject responses from four countries.

Kalish, R.A., and S. Moriwaki. "The world of the elderly Asian American."
   J. SOC. ISSUES 29 (1973): 187-209.

Chapter in this special issue shows problems are similar to other elderly
Americans and that Asian elderly have pressing problems from transplanted
social values to very serious generational differences, all of which need understanding.

Leung, W.T.W., R. Rauanheimo, and F.H. Chang. A SELECT BIBLIOG-
   RAPHY OF EAST-ASIAN FOODS AND NUTRITION ARRANGED
   ACCORDING TO SUBJECT MATTER AND AREA. Atlanta, GA: De-
   partment of Health, Education, and Welfare, 1972.

Discusses Burma, Cambodia, China, Taiwan, Hong Kong, Indonesia, Japan,
Korea, Laos, Malaysia, Philippines, Singapore, Thailand, and Vietnam. Subject
matter categories include food composition, supplements, technology, nutrition,
dietary surveys, nutritional status, and food habits. Lists both published and
unpublished materials.

Massachusetts WIC. NUTRITION EDUCATION MATERIALS. Boston, MA:
   Massachusetts Department of Public Health, 1982.

Discusses Vietnamese, Chinese, Cambodian, and Laotian information, includes materials on baby formula, feeding practices, concerns of pregnant women,
and related topics of value to women, infants, and children.

May, J.M., with collaboration of I.S. Jarcho. THE ECOLOGY OF MAL-
   NUTRITION IN THE FAR AND NEAR EAST. New York: Hafner Publishing Co., 1961.

Includes China, Taiwan, Vietnam, Cambodia, Laos, Thailand, Malaysia,
Burma, India, Ceylon, Pakistan, and Afghanistan in the first part of the volume, rest are Middle Eastern counties. General remarks include items on food

resources, diets, adequacy of food resources, and nutritional disease patterns. This is third volume in the STUDIES IN MEDICAL GEOGRAPHY series. See under Black Americans for greater content details.

Maykovich, M.K. "Asian Americans – Quiet Americans." ETHNIC AMER-
    ICAN MINORITIES. Edited by H.A. Johnson. New York: R.R. Bowker
    Co., 1976, pp. 71-132.

Pre- and postwar background on Chinese, Japanese, Filipinos, and Koreans precedes cultural information on social structure, religions, family, and education. Extensive bibliography. Annotations appear for more than 90 films, 80 filmstrips, 80 slide and transparency sets, and audio and video cassettes, as well as numerous graphics items. Annotations for these last include rental/purchase sources.

McCracken, R.D. "Lactose deficiency: An example of dietary evolution."
    CURR. ANTHRO. 12,4-5 (1971): 479-517.

Hypothesizes and reviews a substantial body of medical literature on the theory that prior to animal domestication all humans were lactose deficient. Discusses implications between culture and human gene frequencies. Eighteen comments to the paper follow, with a reply by the author. There are more than 100 citations from leading medical journals.

Miller, C.D., and B. Branthoover. NUTRITIVE VALUES OF SOME HAWAII
    FOODS. Honolulu, HI: Hawaii Agricultural Experiment Station, 1957.

Household units and common measures of foods frequently used by Asians, including average Chinese and Japanese rice bowl amounts.

Muecke, M.A. "Caring for Southeast Asian refugee patients in the USA."
    AMER. J. PUBLIC HEALTH 73 (1983): 431-438.

Concentrates on Cambodian, Laotian, and Vietnamese refugees; reviews their language, religion, and surname characteristics as well as those of the Hmong, Chinese, and Mien. Discusses the passive and non-compliant patient, body language, and self-care practices. Also explores death and depression comprehension and reaction.

Netland, P.A., and H. Brownstein. "Acculturation and the diet of Asian-
    American elderly." J. NUTR. ELDERLY 3,3 (1984): 37-56.

Majority of subjects of Asian descent in this study of 340 non-institutionalized Asians and Causasians are Chinese (42%) or Japanese (16%). Racial differences include frequency of meals and snacks, use of vitamin supplements, dietary deficiencies, and language and marital profiles. Asians are, as one example of the results indicate, more likely to avoid fatty foods although the intake of cholesterol and the ratio of unsaturated to saturated fatty acids does not vary according to race.

Netland, P.A., and H. Brownstein. "Anthropometric measurements for Asian and Caucasian elderly." J. AMER. DIETET. ASSOC. 85 (1985): 221-223.

Sample of 339 Asians and Caucasians in California reveals similarities in skin-fold measurements and prevalence of obesity.

Orr, K.J. ABOUT HAWAIIAN FOODS AND ANCIENT FOOD CUSTOMS. Honolulu, HI: University of Hawaii Cooperative Extension Service, 1981.

Includes four recipes on staple foods, cooking, ancient and modern customs, and poi making in this polyglot Asian culture.

Peck, R.E., M. Chuang, G.E. Robbins, and M.Z. Nichaman. "Nutritional status of Southeast Asian refugee children." AMER. J. PUBLIC HEALTH 71 (1981): 1144-1148.

Compares 821 children under six arriving in the United States 1979-1980 to those arriving earlier, finds them highly aenemic and stunted compared to the reference group.

Pian, C. ASIAN AMERICAN REFERENCE DATA DIRECTORY. Washington, DC: Office of Asian American Affairs, 1976.

Abstracts of over 480 references relate to health, education, and social welfare characteristics of all Asian populations.

Pickwell, S. "Health screening for Indochinese refugees." NURSE PRACT. 8,4 (1983): 20-25.

Basic screening procedures appropriate for refugees from Southeast Asia and the rationale for their use include health and developmental history, complete physical, vision, and audiometric testing, blood, urine, fecal, and X-ray work.

Rosanoff, A., and D.H. Calloway. "Calcium source in Indochinese immigrants." N. ENG. J. MED. 306,4 (1982): 239-240.

Traditional practices of soaking bones in vinegar reveals appreciable calcium source; tested material yields 120mg in one tablespoon.

Ross Laboratories. NUTRITION MATERIALS. Columbus, OH: Ross Educational Services, 1982.

Series of materials for breast and bottle feeding available in many languages, including Laotian, Hmong, Cambodian, Vietnamese, Korean, Chinese, and Japanese. Many other items available in English and Spanish on other topics.

Santopietro, M.C.S., and D.J. del Bueno. "How to get through to a refugee patient." REG. NURSE (January 1981): 43-46.

Gives tips on how to get help and how to work with an interpreter, addresses for agencies servicing Indochinese refugees; includes a very basic listing of Vietnamese vocabulary for interviewing patients.

Sutherland, J.E., R.F. Avant, W.B. Franz, III, C.M. Monzon, and N.M. Stark. "Indochinese refugee health assessment and treatment." J. FAM. PRAC. 16,1 (1983): 61-67.

Mayo clinic doctors and nurse review data from 426 refugees and note that 17% of the adults have psychological problems, 82% have intestinal parasites, tuberculosis testing is positive in 54%, hepatitus antigen is positive in 13%, hematologic genetic disorders account for most of the 25% incidence of microcytosis, and 80% of the women choose some method of contraception.

Tong, A. "Refugees and the need to understand their problems." J. HOME ECON. (Winter 1981): 21-23.

Addresses refugees' food patterns in America, when healthy, pregnant, or ill. Comparison of consumption of meats, fruits and vegetables of 50 Vietnamese refugees shows little difference in meat consumption at breakfast and increase in use of juice. Lunch changes include use of hamburgers and hot dogs in place of previous intake of fish and shrimp and decrease in green vegetable, cabbage, and pineapple use while doubling orange use. Supper again shows significant decrease in shrimp, bananas, pineapple, and increase in consumption of oranges.

United States Department of Agriculture. "Southeast Asian American nutrition education materials." Washington, DC: Food and Nutrition Service, 1980-1982.

Packet contains six background information folders on nutritional status, tips, use of WIC foods, other materials, sources, and 11 nutrition education handouts in English and Vietnamese – one of these also in Laotian, most on topics related to WIC and with illustrations, one lists spices and foods.

United States Department of Education. BIBLIOGRAPHY. Kansas City, MO: Region VII Refugees Materials Center, 1983.

Several series of materials include hundreds of items for each ethnic group: Vietnamese, Cambodian, Laotian, Chinese, Thai, Korean, and general Asian. Topics include holiday explanations, folkloric materials, health, and employment. Most are free; sources available in this very extensive collection of more than 180 pages of materials.

United States Department of Education. MEDICAL GUIDE AND GLOSSARY. Portland, OR: Indochinese Language Resource Center, n.d.

Manuals are available in English, Laotian, or Vietnamese and contain an introduction to the American health care system. Includes information for specific medical problems and glossary.

Wagner, C., and J. Rullo. MEDICAL GUIDE AND GLOSSARY. Portland, OR: Indochinese Language Resource Center, 1980.

English, Laotian, Vietnamese, and Cambodian editions available that discuss going to the doctor, parts of the body, phrases to describe pain, symptoms, injury, and states of being. Discusses common diseases, medications, immunization, reproductive concerns, preventive health, first aid, a glossary, bibliography, and places to obtain additional information. The foreign language editions are 80 to 150 pages, they have some English to enable one to find equivalent materials.

Wang, H.L. "Tofu and tempeh as potential protein sources in the western diet." J. AMER. OIL CHEM. SOC. 61 (1984): 528-534.

Discusses manufacturing methods, coagulants used for tofu, mold use for tempeh and other oriental fermented and non-fermented soybean foods, with character of resulting products. Also considers their current uses and trends in Asian and non-Asian populations.

Wenlock, R.W., and D.H. Buss. "Nutritional quality of food purchased by Asian families participating in the National Food Survey." PROC. NUTR. SOC. 36,1 (1977): 61A.

British survey results of 21,452 households, identifies 47 Asian households by purchase of flour, rice, onions, dried pulses, butter, or other fats, which are above the normal range. Overall intake of these Asians, ethnicity not identified, was lower than national average for riboflavin and vitamins A and D.

Wilson, J.L., J. Brunson, and M. Johnson. "Health problems of Indo-Chinese immigrants." J. FAM. PRAC. 12 (1981): 551-557.

Family practice conference session is setting for discussion of problems of Laotian family, agency report on refugee resettlement problems, and protocol developed for dealing with health problems. Details tuberculosis, immunizations, malaria, hepatitus, leprosy, venereal diseases, and intestinal parasites with symptoms observed and recommendations for screening.

Wong, H.B. "Rice water in the treatment of infantile gastroenteritis." LANCET 2,8237 (1981): 102-103.

Compares oral electrolyte solution and rice water as dilutant with milk in hospitalized infants. Rice water mixture reduces number of stools and some indications are that the rice water's lower osmolality reduces the risk of increasing intestinal secretion.

Yu, E.S., and B.K. Cypress. "Visits to physicians by Asian Pacific Americans." MED. CARE 20 (1982): 809-820.

Discusses findings of the 1979 National Ambulatory Medical Care Survey. These include no significant differences between Asian/Pacific Islanders and Whites with regard to return visit ratio, diagnostics taken, and services rendered. Other findings are, that children are major users of ambulatory medical care among Asian/Pacific Americans, that they visit physicians less, and that more visits by Thai populations are made for preventive care. Includes cultural reasons for these findings.

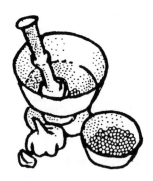

6.10   Asian Resources for Recipes

6.10.1   Indonesian

Though not listed separately in the introductory section, some Asians coming to the United States pass through and/or are influenced by the islands of the archipelago of Indonesia where Chinese, Indian, Arab, and Dutch influences abound.

DeWit, A., and A. Borghese. THE COMPLETE BOOK OF INDONESIAN COOKING. New York: Bobbs-Merrill Company, 1973.

Background material discusses region, foods, and spices indigenous to these islands and how to use them. Ingredient list tells how to pronounce what they are, and where they may be purchased. Recipe chapters begin with details of the item, which may be be it rijsttafel, sate, other meats, sayurs, or sambals. All are carefully explained.

Johns, Y. DISHES FROM INDONESIA. Philadelphia, PA: Chilton Book Co., 1971.

Background materials detail preparation techniques and ingredients. Chapters are arranged according to main ingredient and begin with introductory food item information. Full page color photographs illustrate some dozen dishes.

Marks, C., and M. Soeharjo. THE INDONESIAN KITCHEN. New York: Atheneum, 1981.

Recipes are prepared for the American kitchen and include island of origin. Introductory material is limited to items needed for food preparation. Glossary includes ingredients and their Latin names.

Owen, S. INDONESIAN FOOD AND COOKERY. London: Prospect Books, 1976.

Originally published as THE HOME BOOK OF INDONESIAN COOKERY, this expanded volume has several additional sections and more material in the revised sections. The 88-page introduction and glossary are extensive as they detail customs, food behaviors, cookery techniques, and ingredients. Recipes, arranged according to main ingredient, begin with a short introduction and are detailed.

128 *Other Asian Americans*

6.10.2   Korean

Hyun, J. THE KOREAN COOKBOOK. Chicago: Follett Publishing Co., 1970.

Background information includes some history, meal patterns, home life, ingredients and their use, and techniques helpful in preparation. Recipes, by the main ingredient, often begin with introductory material. Glossary of ingredients.

6.10.3   Laotian

Davidson, A. FISH AND FISH DISHES OF LAOS. Rutland, VT: Charles E. Tuttle Co., 1975.

Begins with a catalogue of local fish, illustrating each and detailing size, name in several countries in the region, and information about use in Laotian cuisine. This is thorough and encompasses the first half of the book. Second half has glossary of equipment and ingredients, each illustrated. The recipes follow, many with short introductions. Last chapter has additional recipes from neighboring countries of Burma, Thailand, Cambodia, and Vietnam. A bibliography follows.

Sing, P. TRADITIONAL RECIPES OF LAOS. London: Prospect Books, 1981.

This is edited translation of two of the recipe books by the late Phia Sing, chef of the Royal Palace at Luang Prabang. Text begins with Laotian eating habits, attitudes towards food, and their significances. Culinary terms and equipment are detailed. The recipes follow with original hand-written copy on the left and English translation of ingredients followed by the method of preparation on the right. A chapter of Laotian desserts is added. Bibliography is of books consulted; many pertain to foods and cuisines of the region. Bilingual index.

6.10.4   Malaysian

Hitchcock, J., editor. THE FLAVOUR OF SINGAPORE. London: Four Corners Publishing Co., 1973.

This volume on Singapore cookery features recipes from restaurants. They are Malay, Chinese, Nonya, and European. Many color photographs illustrate the finished dishes.

Lee, C.K. MRS. LEE'S COOKBOOK. Singapore: Eurasia Press, 1974.

This collection of Nonya food includes a few of the author's favorite Singaporean and Chinese dishes. There are a few color plates and a glossary of ingredients translated into Malay, Chinese characters, Indonesian, Thai, Indian script, Tagalong, with the botanical name for the local items. (Nonya, also called Peranakan, is a blending of Chinese and Malay food.)

Leong, Y.S. THE ART OF ORIENTAL COOKING. London: Andre Deutsch Limited, 1977.

A short glossary and introduction precedes the recipes for Nonya and western cakes, other desserts, Singaporean favorites, and Nonya appetizers, meat, poultry, seafood, rice and noodles, soups, and vegetable and pickle selections. Many color plates.

6.10.5   Thai

Brennan, J. THE ORIGINAL THAI COOKBOOK. New York: Richard Marek Publishers, 1981.

Extensive introduction includes background and culture of the cuisine, a blend of Chinese, Indian, and Arabic influences. Details Thai kitchens and equipment and use of basic ingredients. Recipes are by main ingredient. Each chapter begins with regional material. There is a glossary of food words, with detailed cultural and explanatory information about most of them. A long list of sources follows.

Kritakara, M.L.T., and M.R.P. Amranand. MODERN THAI COOKING. Bangkok, Thailand: Duang Kamol Editions, 1977.

Introduction includes some background and an extensive glossary of ingredients with food names in English, Thai script, and phonetics; each is illustrated. Recipes are given as twelve monthly menus and are written in both languages. Color photographs illustrate many of the recipes; introduction to customs precedes each chapter.

Pinsuvana, M. COOKING THAI FOOD IN AMERICAN KITCHENS. Bangkok, Thailand: Sahamitr Industrial Printing, 1976.

Spiral bound format contains recipes in both English and Thai. Almost all recipes with photograph of completed dish. Sections by main food or meal item.

Schmitz, P.C., and M.J. Worman. PRACTICAL THAI COOKING. Tokyo,
Japan: Kodansha International, 1985.

Recipes for basic items such as sauces, pastes, and dips precede main food
ingredient chapters. Each of these begins with small amount of cultural material.
Extensive list of ingredient sources. Some color plates.

6.10.6   Vietnamese

Miller, J.N.H. VIETNAMESE COOKERY. Rutland, VT: Charles E. Tuttle
Co., 1968.

Introductory material and glossary of ingredients, many with possible sub-
titutes if unavailable, followed by recipes in main ingredient or meal item categories.

Ngo, B., and G. Zimmerman. THE CLASSIC CUISINE OF VIETNAM.
Woodbury, NY: Barron's Educational Series, 1979.

Introduction, equipment, and ingredient glossary with some storage informa-
tion precedes some basic ingredient recipes and a chapter on traditional favorites.
Recipes by main ingredient headings follow as does a menu planning chapter.
Photographs illustrate some techniques, some mail order food sources follow.

6.10.7   Mixed Southeast Asian

The following volumes indicate countries where recipes are divided by country.
Unless introductory material is extensive, it is not mentioned. Indicated also
are some other features of note.

Anwar, Z. WITH AN EASTERN FLAVOR. Singapore: MPH Distributers,
1978.

Recipes of Indonesia, North India, South India, and Singapore. Color photographs of local spices; includes a food glossary.

Brennan, J. THE CUISINES OF ASIA. New York: St. Martin's/Marek,
1984.

Recipes by technique, not country. Detailed background on countries and
cuisines of China, India, Indonesia, Japan, Korea, Malaysia and Singapore, the
Philippines, Thailand, and Vietnam.

Brissenden, R. ASIA'S UNDISCOVERED CUISINE. New York: Pantheon Books, 1970.

Originally published as SOUTH-EAST ASIAN FOOD by Penguin Books, the recipes are from Indonesia, Malaysia and Singapore, and Thailand. Glossary of ingredients and cross-country list of food items with names in English, Indonesian, Malay, Hindustani and Tamil, Cantonese, and Thai.

Buck, P.S. ORIENTAL COOKBOOK. New York: Simon and Schuster, 1972.

Recipes from Thailand, Burma, India-Pakistan, China, the Philippines, Indochina, Korea, Malaysia, and Japan. Glossary and mail-order sources.

Conil, J., and D. MacCarthy. ORIENTAL COOKERY. London: Croom Helm, 1978.

Recipes from China, Hong Kong, Taiwan, Japan, Korea, Vietnam, Cambodia, Thailand, Malaysia, Singapore, Burma, Indonesia, Philippines, India, and Pakistan.

Dorje, R. FOOD IN TIBETAN LIFE. London: Prospect Books, 1985.

Detailed introduction about the country, people, festivals, social customs, and food. Recipes are detailed and include background information. Source material and glossary in English, Tibetan script, and phonetics in two different transcriptions.

Horsting, M., F. de Lannoy, J. Davis, and L. Cao. FLAVORS OF SOUTH-EAST ASIA. San Francisco, CA: 101 Productions, 1979.

Recipes from Indonesia, Thailand, and Vietnam. Mail-order sources and glossary.

Howe, R. FAR EASTERN COOKERY. London: International Wine and Food Publishing Co., 1969.

Recipes from India, Pakistan, Kashmir, Nepal, Ceylon, Burma, Thailand, Malaysia, Singapore, Indonesia, Cambodia, Vietnam, China, Japan, Korea, and the Philippines. Glossary included.

Khiang, M.M. COOK AND ENTERTAIN THE BURMESE WAY. Ann Arbor, MI: Karoma Publishers, 1978.

Details background of Burmese cooking, food customs, and includes recipes divided into food categories.

Laas, W., editor. CUISINES OF THE EASTERN WORLD. New York: Golden Press, 1967.

Recipes from China, Japan, and the "World of Curry," which includes India, Indonesia, Thailand, and Malaysia, and others. Considerable background material, some cross-cultural, has color plates.

Moore, I., and J. Godfrey, editors. THE COMPLETE ORIENTAL COOKBOOK. London: Marshall Cavendish Books, 1978.

Recipes from China, India, Japan, and Southeast Asia. Many color photographs.

Ng, D. COMPLETE ASIAN MEALS. Singapore: Times Books International, 1979.

Recipes are Malay and Indonesian, Chinese, Nonya (Peranakan), Indian, and Sri Lankan. Color photographs of some recipes, packaged foods, Asian vegetables, and spices. Glossary of ingredients in English, Malay, and Chinese characters.

Piper, M.R., editor. SUNSET ORIENTAL COOKBOOK. Menlo Park, CA: Lane Books, 1970.

Recipes from China, Japan, and Korea. Background material on Oriental food as an art. Information on shopping, utensils, ingredients, and menu planning.

Schryver, A. ORIENTAL COOKING. New York: Grosset & Dunlap, 1975.

Recipes from China, Japan, and Korea. Glossary and mail-order sources.

Solomon, C. THE COMPLETE ASIA COOKBOOK. New York: McGraw-Hill Book Co., 1976.

Recipes from India and Pakistan, Sri Lanka, Indonesia, Malaysia, Singapore, Burma, Thailand, Cambodia and Laos, Vietnam, the Philippines, China, Korea, and Japan. Extensive glossary with names of the items in the languages of the countries of use, botanical names included.

THREE HUNDRED ASIAN BEST RECIPES. Hong Kong: Vista Productions, 1979.

Recipes from Indonesia, the Philippines, Singapore, Malaysia, Thailand, Burma, Korea, Vietnam, Cambodia, Laos, China, Japan, India, Sri Lanka, and Pakistan. Color photograph of each.

Waldo, M. THE COMPLETE BOOK OF ORIENTAL COOKING. New York: Bantam Books, 1960.

Recipes from Hawaii and the islands of the Pacific, Japan, Korea, Philippines, Indonesia, China, Malaya, Thailand, Burma, and India.

Wright, J., editor. THE ENCYCLOPEDIA OF ASIAN COOKING. London: Octopus Books Limited, 1980.

Recipes from India, Pakistan, Bangladesh, Malaysia, Singapore, Indonesia, Burma, Thailand, Kampuchea, Laos, Vietnam, China, Japan, the Philippines, and Korea. Measurements in metric and American measures; has glossary and many color photographs.

Chapter 7

INDIAN AMERICANS

7.1 Introduction

Indian cuisines are unusual and varied, a reflection of the differences that abound
from one province to the next and include language, food habits, cooking methods, and even the style of wearing the sari. These plus differences in culture and
religion and the climate of this large country greatly influence the cuisines.

In northern India, wheat is the primary grain and breads such as chapatis,
parathas, and naan are the staple foods. There are many elaborate meat dishes,
cooked in a clarified butter called ghee. Hot spiced tea is the favorite drink of
the cold winters. Also in the north, tandoori baked dishes are common as are
kabobs, biryonis or meat and rice combination dishes with nuts and saffron, and
milk based Bengali sweets.

In the south where people enjoy freshly roasted coffee, rice is the staple grain
served throughout the meal whose dishes are more highly spiced than those in
the north. Many people from southern India are vegetarians and they have
a well-developed meatless culinary repertoire. Large quantities of coconut oil
and milk are used and idles (steamed rice cakes) and dosas, which are rice and
lentils with chutney, are popular dishes. The people in the south prefer steamed
to baked foods.

In India, "curry" is any dish with a richly spiced sauce that is very carefully
cooked to blend all of the spices together with the flavors of the meat, fish,
and/or vegetables. The curry may be complex or simple, depending upon the
addition of other flavors. These may be onions, garlic, ginger, tomatoes, coconut,
nuts, and/or yogurt. The Indian cook grinds spices daily and every spice added
to a particular dish is carefully chosen for its individual flavor. It is this delicate
art of spicing, the use of cumin, coriander, turmeric, chilis, ginger, cinnamon,

mustard seeds, cardamom, fenugreek, and other spices, that creates the Indian cuisine. Due to limited refrigeration facilities the people of India discovered that foods cooked in certain spices would not spoil easily.

Indians use large amounts of cereals and legumes, fairly large amounts of dairy products, and smaller amounts of vegetables and fruits, many of these as pickles, chutneys, or condiments. Meat and fish are used in even lesser amounts and only by those who are affluent and are not vegetarians. Some Hindu vegetarians do eat fish. They consider them fruits of the sea. Sweets are commonplace for all. They are very sweet by American standards.

The majority of Indians eat two main meals a day with the early morning one offering wheat or rice and coffee or tea laced with sugar and boiled milk, the choice dependent on particular regions. Sometimes fruit or pickles are served at this meal, in the evening meal they are always present. Rice and dahl, which are lentils, are served at the evening meal along with some curried vegetables, and if consumed, meat or meat and rice. This meal usually ends with a very sweet milk based dessert and sometimes a yogurt or buttermilk beverage.

India has a high prevalence of protein-calorie malnutrition (PCM). Cultural traditions remain and dictate that women feed the breadwinner of the family and the children first, even if they, the women, are malnourished or ill. In India, the maternal death rate, incidence of stillbirths, and low birth weight of infants are high. Many Indian children suffer PCM, vitamin A and vitamin B deficiencies, and iron and folacin deficiency anemias.

There is significant improvement in the nutritional status of Indians who emigrate to the United States or are second or later generation Americans. Many of their traditional food beliefs continue and some of these include the discarding of colostrum and/or not feeding a newborn until the third day of life, the late introduction of solid foods, dilution of milk, and fasting, often for long periods of time. Research has shown that Indian women introduce their babies to soft rice at six months. It is the only solid food given and is provided four times a day.

Many Indian immigrants continue to follow vegetarian regimens and their protein, iron, and vitamin B_{12} intake may be marginal. The overall diet tends to have up to 26% of the total calories from fat sources compared to the American national average of 40%.

With dietary changes have come increased risk of developing coronary heart disease, hypertension, gastro-intestinal tract disorders, and to a lesser degree, obesity. Most Indian women report respiratory infections, gastro-intestinal tract disorders, and measles as high on their list of health concerns.

Improvement in the diet would be reduction in the use of sweeteners and increase in the use of fresh fruits and vegetables, particularly the green leafy ones. Recommendations include additional sources of iron, more foods with complex carbohydrates, and others high in the B vitamins.

For nutrient analysis of foods specific to their diet, see the Tables of Food Composition.

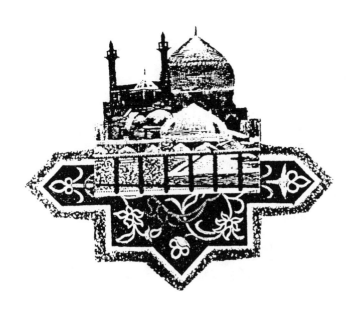

7.2   References

Abraham, R. "Trace element intake by Asians during pregnancy." PROC. NUTR. SOC. 41,2 (1982): 261-265.

Seven-day dietary intake of Asians, 20 of whom are vegetarians, 20 non-vegetarians, and non-Asians are assessed and copper levels in all groups are below standards set by health department. Zinc intakes are substantially lower in the vegetarian group. Phytic acid and dietary fiber intakes are higher in the Asians, thus incidence of these trace elements are considerably less for the vegetarians. Asians in this study are all of Indian descent.

Attariwala, R. "Asian children and school meals in the UK – A question of choice." J. HUMAN NUTR. 31 (1977): 251-255.

Article begins by reviewing meal patterns and foods of Asians of Indian descent. Five percent of the school children in this study are in the category of poorly fed. When given a choice, 62.5% select a snack instead of the main lunch meal.

Balasubramaniam, G. "Modifications of indigenous food habits of Indians currently residing in Columbus, Ohio." Ph.D. dissertation. Ohio State University, 1976.

Study identifies greater frequency of consumption of non-vegetarian foods, commercially prepared breads, breakfast cereals, cheeses, carbonated beverages, and fruits in the United States than in India, and observes decrease in use of rice, unleavened wheat breads, yogurt, vegetables, dried legumes, and beans. Fewer meals are prepared at home in the United States, and many do not consume Indian meals daily.

Banerjee, S., and B. Pal. "Zinc content of foodstuffs." INDIAN J. NUTR. DIETET. 16 (1979): 320-325.

Gives mean values for 122 cereals, pulses, roots, tubers, vegetables, spices, condiments, fruits, animal products, dairy foods, and miscellaneous items.

Banik, N.D.D., S. Nayar, R. Krishna, S. Bakshi, and A.D. Taskar. "Growth period of Indian school children in relation to nutrition and adolescence." INDIAN J. PEDIAT. 40 (1973): 173-179.

Children from well-privileged groups compare with 50th percentile of American standard for weight, height and arm and calf circumferences. Underprivileged children correspond with the 10th percentile of the American standard.

The time of the adolescent growth spurt varies depending on the nutritional status of the child; it is later in the underprivileged.

Bose, T. "High dietary fiber in routine Bengalee diet." INDIAN J. NUTR. DIETET. 16 (1979): 312-319.

Typical diet is very high in fiber. Both diabetic and normal subjects show significant changes when this diet is followed. Normal group is less prone to hyperglycemia and some diabetics are able to discontinue medication after using this diet.

Brown, K.H., M. Khatin, and M.G. Ahmed. "Relationship of the xylose absorption status of children in Bangladesh to their absorption of macronutrients from local diets." AMER. J. CLIN. NUTR. 34 (1981): 1540-1547.

Study of 31 asymptomatic Bangladeshi children concludes that the diminished absorption of xylose does not necessarily indicate impaired absorption and tropical enteropathy may not have major nutritional significance for those individuals with manifestations of the syndrome.

Brown, K.H., L. Parry, M. Khatun, and M.G. Ahmed. "Lactose malabsorption in Bangladeshi village children: Relation with age, history of recent diarrhea, nutritional status, and breast feeding." AMER. J. CLIN. NUTR. 32 (1979): 1962-1969.

By means of hydrogen breath test diagnoses lactose malabsorption found in 80% of the children over age three, but none in those under six months. A large number of children with acute signs of undernutrition have signs of malabsorption.

Ferro-Luzzi, G.E. "Ritual as language: The case of South Indian food offerings." CURR. ANTHRO. 18 (1977): 507-514.

Food offerings and their ethnographic context show them to be an expression of love. Many are given in pairs, the number five is the culturally most favored number, three also important as specific food offerings use contrasting combinations, all with special meaning.

Ganapathy, S., and R. Dhanda. "Protein and iron nutrition in lacto-ovo-vegetarian Indo-Aryan United States residents." INDIAN J. NUTR. DIETET. 17 (1980): 45-52.

North Indians or Punjabis studying in the United States maintain their lacto-ovo vegetarian diets. Nitrogen intake for a seven-day period offers a negative nitrogen balance. Iron consumption is adequate. Table with food pattern of the diet for the seven-day period shows items but not amounts consumed.

Ganapathy, S., and R. Dhanda. "Selenium content of omnivorous and vegetarian diets." INDIAN J. NUTR. DIETET. 16 (1979): 53-55.

Analyzes serving portions of college cafeteria omnivorous diet, a home-cooked lacto-ovo vegetarian diet, and a laboratory administered all vegetable diet for seven days for selenium and finds mean results of 93, 82, and 86 micrograms per day, respectively.

Gans, B. "The nutritional status of West Indian immigrants." PROC. NUTR. SOC. 26 (1967): 218-222.

Finds instances of suboptimal nutrition frequently after the first six months of life. Iron deficiency anemia at the toddler stage is common, hookworm infestation is difficult to assess, and by school entry age hemoglobin levels are usually normal for those born in the United Kingdom. Other nutritional deficiencies result in rickets, lack of fluoride, prurutic skin lesions, and borderline cases of hypoalbuminemia.

Gupta, S.P. "Changes in the food habits of Asian Indians in the United States, a case study." SOC. SOCIAL. RES. 60 (1975): 87-99.

Acculturation proceeds in three phases as the amount of interaction with the host society increases. Items of importance in decreasing value are marital status, age, sex, length of stay, caste, and rural-urban background.

Hasan, K.A. "The Hindu dietary and culinary practices in a North Indian village: An ethnomedical and structural analysis." ETHNOMEDIZIN 1 (1971): 43-69.

Investigates foods and the seasonal cycle, methods of cooking, foods consumed during various stages of the life cycle, restrictions, taboos, dichotomy of hot and cold, and shows that quantity and quality are only important when recommending strengthening foods.

Hunt, S. "Traditional Asian food customs." J. HUMAN NUTR. 31 (1977): 245-248.

Food habits vary depending on region of origin. Article discusses Punjabis, Mirpuris, Gujaratis, Pakistanis, and Bengalis in terms of their regional variations, religious food prohibitions, and nutrient deficiencies. The latter can include vitamin D and B_{12} deficiencies, folate, and iron shortfalls.

Khan, M.A., and B.O. Eggum. "The nutritive value of some Pakistani diets."
J. SCI. FD. AGRIC. 29 (1978): 1023-1029.

Chemical analysis of diets reveals 13% of total calories from protein, 61% from carbohydrates, and 11% from fat. Lysine and threonine are limiting amino acids in the national diet but protein is not Three meals a day are usually eaten in Pakistan.

Khan-Siddiqui, L., and M.S. Bamji. "Plasma carnitine levels in adult males in India: Effects of high cereal, low fat diet, fat supplementation, and nutritional status." AMER. J. CLIN. NUTR. 33 (1980): 1259-1263.

Apparently healthy subjects consuming predominantly cereal based diets have normal levels of plasma carnitine and albumin. Subjects with evidence of malnutrition and normal albumin have higher plasma carnitine levels. Increases of dietary fat reduce plasma carnitine markedly and raise acyl carnitine. Results suggest levels of plasma carnitine may be regulated by a balance between factors influencing its availability or its synthesis, and utilization.

Khare, R.S. THE HINDO HEARTH AND HOME. New Delhi, India: Vikas Publishing House, 1976.

An ethnographic look at contemporary ways of handling foods in North Indian households with culinary relations and meanings. Food areas, cooking, serving, eating, ceremonial feasts and features and implications of each included.

Lannoy, R. THE SPEAKING TREE, A STUDY OF INDIAN CULTURE AND SOCIETY. New York: Oxford University Press, 1971.

Several of the five parts in this volume discuss relationship of children and parents, status of women, sexuality, attitudes in general, and marital relations and roles. Provides understanding of interpersonal relationships.

MacPhail, A.P., T.H. Bothwell, J.D. Torrance, D.P. Derman, W.R. Bezwoda, R.W. Charlton, and F.G.H. Mayet. "Iron nutrition in Indian women at different ages." SOUTH AFRICAN MED. J. 59 (1981): 939-942.

Iron status of 320 Indian women living in South Africa reveals 14% prevalence of anemia. An additional 26% have depleted iron stores. Measurements of iron are higher in older women and there is evidence that the duration of menstruation has a significant effect on iron status.

McKensie, J.C., and P. Mumford. "Food habits of West Indian immigrants."
PROC. NUTR. SOC. 34 (1964): xlii-xliii.

Most families quickly adopt some English foods, mostly snack items and breakfast foods. Of the main meals eaten at home, 85% have West Indian foods. This adherence of dinner custom continues among those who live in Britain more than five years.

Mudambi, S.R., and M.V. Rajagopal. FUNDAMENTAL OF FOOD AND NUTRITION. New Delhi, India: Wiley Eastern Ltd., 1981.

Paperback concentrates on nutrition with little space devoted to food science. Appendix has information on food composition of Indian foods and some anthropometric data. Throughout it highlights food and nutrition from Indian cultural perspectives.

Ong, S.P., J. Ryley, T. Bashir, and H.N. MacDonald. "Nutrient intake and associated biochemical status of pregnant Asians in the United Kingdom." HUMAN NUTR.: APP. NUTR. 37A (1983): 23-29.

A comparison of 46 women of Pakistani, Indian, and Bangladeshi origin at eight and twenty weeks of pregnancy indicates that all need more calcium and vitamin D. Those from Bangladesh also need to increase their iron intake. Levels of 25-hydroxycholecalciferol in plasma indicate the importance of food sources of vitamin D.

Rao, C.N., and B.S.N. Rao. "Trace element content of Indian foods and the dietaries." INDIAN J. MED. RES. 73 (1981): 904-909.

Determines magnesium, chromium, copper, manganese, and zinc content of cereals, pulses, vegetables, animal products, and other commonly used foods by atomic absorption spectroscopy. These data are then used to compute typical diets at two income levels typical of seven states of India. Diets are low in copper and zinc and are less well absorbed than is intake in higher income diets.

Robertson, I., B.M. Glenkin, J.B. Henderson, W.B. McIntosh, A. Lakhani, and M.G. Dunnigan. "Nutritional deficiencies among ethnic minorities in the United Kingdom." PROC. NUTR. SOC. 41 (1982): 243-256.

Article indicates that ethnic minorities have origins in West Indies, India, China, and Africa and illustrative material concentrates on the first two of these groups. Major problems include obesity, infantile rickets, iron deficiency anemia, deficiencies of folic acid and vitamin B_{12}. Paper concentrates on the problems of rickets and osteomalacia.

Satyanarayana, K., A.N. Naidu, and B.S.N. Rao. "Nutritional deprivation in childhood and the body size, activity, and physical work capacity of young boys." AMER. J. CLIN. NUTR. 32 (1979): 1769-1775.

Evaluates children ages 14 to 17 for whom there are nutritional status records when they were five years old. Severe undernutrition during childhood has no effect on work performance but these subjects have significantly higher heart rate at moderate work levels.

Storer, J. "Hot and cold food beliefs in an Indian community and their significance." J. HUMAN NUTR. 31 (1977): 33-40.

In interviews about the hot-cold concept, women in 45 Hindu homes reveal that they do not know its origin and that they are not in complete agreement about foods belonging to either of its classifications. Ordinarily, little attention is paid; however, seasonal considerations such as avoidance of green leafy vegetables in winter because they are cold or eggs in summer because they are hot, and implementation of their use in vulnerable stages of life such as pregnancy, lactation, and illness are still practiced.

Tandon, R.K., Y.K. Joshi, D.S. Singh, M. Narendranathan, V. Balakrishnan, and K. Lal. "Lactose intolerance in North and South Indians." AMER. J. CLIN. NUTR. 34 (1981): 943-946.

Indians from the north showed less lactose intolerance (27.4%) than did those from the south (66.6%). Reasons for lower incidence in the north may be that they are descendents of the Aryans who are used to dairy products and are lactose tolerant.

Thanpy, R. "Therapeutic diets for Asians." J. HUMAN NUTR. 31 (1977): 256-258.

Guidance is provided to improve some known deficiencies of some nutrients including vitamins D and B_{12}, folate, and calcium. Gives a 1100 kcal diet and advises for low salt, low fat, and vegetarian diets. A few customs and concerns included.

Thimmayamma, B.V.S., P. Rau, V.K. Desai, and B.N. Jayaprakesh. "A study of changes in socioeconomic conditions, dietary intake and nutritional status of Indian rural families over a decade." ECOL. FD. NUTR. 5 (1976): 235-243.

Only changes have been are increase in income and a small increase in milk consumption but this is offset by increase in prices. Overall, health remains the same. Mean intake of energy and protein is above 90% of Indian Recommended Allowances.

Thomas, P. FESTIVALS AND HOLIDAYS OF INDIA. Bombay, India: D.B. Taraporevala Sons and Co., n.d.

Details Hindu, Muslim, Sikh, tribal, Christian, Buddist, Jains, Parsis, Jewish, national, and secular festivals. Excellent background materials, though not much on foods; cross-cultural information helps clarify similarities and differences.

Wharton, P.A., P.M. Eaton, and K.C. Day. "Sorrento Asian: Food tables, recipes, and customs of mothers attending Sorrento Maternity Hospital, Birmingham, England." HUMAN NUTR.: APP. NUTR. 37A (1983): 378-402.

Muslim, Sikh, and Hindu women reveal meal patterns, cooking methods, and problems encountered when shopping. Differences based on area of origin show considerable variation. Recipes with amounts calculated by weight included. Fasting rites and other beliefs are still practiced and table shows differences by region. Detailed nutrient analysis for 60 foods or dishes.

Ziporyn, T. "Possible link probed: Deafness and vitamin D." J. AMER. MED. ASSOC. 250 (1983): 1951-2015.

Asians in Britain are at particular risk for rickets and osteomalacia because of vitamin D deficiency, 21 patients over age 60 with low or borderline levels of this nutrient show progressive deafness. Some show evidence of cochlear demineralization. Six patients are followed long enough to assess response to treatment with calciferol, in four, hearing is improved 10 dB or more.

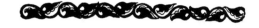

7.3   Resources for Recipes

Items that follow are specific only to India. Others can be found in: Other Asian Resources for Recipes.

Chowdhary, S. INDIAN COOKING. London: Andre Deutsch, 1954.

Introductory section includes materials on basic ingredients and instructions on how to make several. Recipes are in main ingredient chapters with heavy emphasis on vegetables, pulses, breads, and sweets.

Collins, R.P. A WORLD OF CURRIES. New York: Avenel Books, 1967.

Most recipes are from India and Pakistan, a few from China, Indonesia, South Africa, and Australia; they are not so indicated. Glossary of spices includes botanical names.

Dalal, T. INDIAN VEGETARIAN COOKBOOK. New York: St. Martin's Press, 1985.

Short introduction includes kitchen equipment and menus. Recipes are by main ingredient or meal item and each chapter has some general information. Short glossary and a few color plates.

Dandakar, V. SALADS OF INDIA. Trumansburg, NY: The Crossing Press, 1983.

Recipes divided by main salad ingredient, each preceded by short cultural commentary.

Dandekar, H.C. BEYOND CURRY. Ann Arbor, MI: Center for Southeast Asian Studies of the University of Michigan, 1983.

A range of Indian dishes, most meatless, are divided by meal item or main ingredient. They feature cuisine of the Maharashtra State on the west coast of India.

Jaffrey, M. MADHUR JAFFREY'S INDIAN COOKING. Woodbury, NY: Barrons, 1980.

Chapters on technique, seasonings, and menu planning with the recipes and color photographs of about one-quarter of the completed dishes. Some background materials.

Lal, P. INDIAN COOKING FOR PLEASURE. London: Hamlyn Publishing
   Group, 1970.

   Recipes in chapters by main ingredients. Each chapter has small amount of
introductory food or culture use.

Rau, S.R. THE COOKING OF INDIA. New York: Time-Life Books, 1969.

   Detailed background on the culture and foods of India with a chapter on
neighboring Pakistan and Bangladesh; all discuss roots and current practices.
Recipes also appear in companion volume RECIPES: THE COOKING OF IN-
DIA; neither indicates regionality.

Sahni, J. CLASSIC INDIAN VEGETARIAN AND GRAIN COOKING. New
   York: William Morrow Co., 1985.

   Extensive glossary on ingredients and equipment in first hundred pages.
Recipes are by main ingredient or meal item and most include cultural information. Extensive list of ingredient and equipment sources.

Sharma, P.V. FRUITS AND VEGETABLES IN ANCIENT INDIA. Varanasi,
   India: Chaukhambha Orientalia, 1979.

   Introduction emphasizes historical, medical, and current importance given
to fruits and vegetables. Includes list of English, Latin, Sanskrit, and Hindi
names.

Singh, M.S. THE SPICE BOX. Trumansburg, NY: The Crossing Press, 1981.

   Vegetarian cookbook with recipes divided by main ingredient and each chapter introduction discusses their place in the diet.

Stendahl. THE BOMBAY PALACE COOKBOOK. NEW YORK: Dodd,
   Mead and Co., 1985.

   Recipes from Bombay Palace restaurant represent Moghlai cookery of the
north, they follow background materials.

Chapter 8

MIDDLE EASTERN AMERICANS AND SOME FROM THE MEDITERRANEAN

8.1 Introduction

Cultural and culinary interaction abound around the Mediterranean Sea. Despite a long history of political strife and conquest, food ideas have crossed national boundaries to become blended and reborn in other cultures. Culinary traditions do vary from country to country, but there are many more similarities than differences, especially among Arabian neighbors.

When discussing the foods of the region, it is appropriate to think of things culinary in terms of certain flavors and tastes: the fresh aromas of wild herbs, the tang of lemons and oranges, the texture of olives and dates, and the combination of garlic and oil, or the mix of honey and nuts. Tomatoes, peppers, eggplants, chick peas, lentils and beans, yogurt and cheese, pasta, couscous, and figs are the foods of the region.

The chick peas, lentils, and beans that have been cultivated since farming first began are used in many ways by many of the people with roots in this region. Eggplants brought to the area fifteen hundred years ago took root. They are now prepared in all of the cultures in hundreds of ways. Olives are found everywhere and are, according to legend, Athena's "gift of plenty." They are used whole, are essential as oil, and as such are used in combination with garlic. Herbs and spices are also important. Many of them and many of the other seasonings, such as the mints, orange and rose waters, mastic, oregano, chili peppers, and lemon juice, are used to awaken sluggish appetites.

8.2   Greek

Bread, olives, fruits, nuts, and legumes are diet staples. Vegetables are common, and meats, if affordable, are most often lamb or chicken. Affordable or not, they are always served for feast days. Milk drinking is rare but use of dairy products is not. Yogurt is very popular as are cheeses, the most famous of which is the Greek feta cheese. It is semi-soft, crumbly, salty, and made from goat's milk. It is used extensively in cooking and in salads. In the latter, it appears at every dinner meal. Desserts are very sweet, as is coffee, served Turkish style, strong and laced with sugar. Both are popular at lunch and dinner, and at the frequent daily snack times.

8.3   Italian

Italy is divided by a north-south gastronomic boundary referred to as the pasta line, the cooking fats line, the coffee line, the meats line, or the poverty line. None is accurate but a striking division is the pasta line, the country's universal food, which in the north is most often flat and limp and in the south stiff, brittle, and usually made without egg. The north is dairy country where butter, eggs, and cream are used extensively along with wheat as the primary grain and polenta popular, too. In the south, olive oil predominates for cooking and salad use, wheat use also predominates, but creamy sauces are less popular. Sauces made with tomato are the rule. Meat, milk, sugar, and wine consumption is higher among northerers and bread, fish, and pasta consumption higher among southerners. Overall the protein for both is stable, fat use has doubled, and carbohydrate intake increases are about 25%, yielding a mean intake of many more calories.

8.4   Saudi Arabian

Flat breads along with legumes are staples in this predominantly vegetarian cuisine. Meats are used, if affordable. Pork is forbidden to those of the Muslim faith as is shellfish, the predominant meat is lamb, the next most popular chicken. These are always served on feast days. Onions, leeks, and tomatoes are popular vegetables and they are served alone or with eggplants and legumes. Fruits are not consumed very often, nor is milk. Tea and coffee are popular and served very sweet;these and huge quantities of food are served to all guests as signs of hospitality.

8.5 Iranian

In this land of mild but aromatic seasonings, lamb is again the favorite meat. With a large Muslim population, pork and seafood use is rare. Rice is served at most meals; fruits are common in cooking and used for desserts. Many other sweets are also served. Snacks are popular and they, too, are often very sweet. Coffee may be served but it is rarely sweet; tea when used is always served sweet.

8.6 Lebanese, Syrian, Jordanian, and Iraqi

These cuisines are quite similar and enjoy okra, eggplant, and squash and citrus fruits along with mostly flat breads, bulgar wheat, yogurt and other soured milks. Lamb is the meat of choice, prepared as are all foods with lots of herbs, garlic, cinnamon, coriander, and mint and with olive oil which is used extensively. Sweets are popular and are very sweet as they usually are in countries with Arabic roots. Holidays, feast days, and fast days vary depending upon individual religions. For instance, the Lebanese have a large Christian population and many are Greek Orthodox. The Syrians are mostly Muslim. An overview of their holidays and others can be found in the references. See Barer-Stein and others in the Mixed Ethnic References, as well.

8.7 Turkish

Breads, usually unleavened, fruits, vegetables, sour milk products, legumes and some fish, lamb, and chicken are staples of a diet that has main meals and many small meals or meza during each day. Sweetened coffee accompanies all of the meals when foods mix Arabic and Western influences.

8.8 Israeli

No clearcut cuisine has emerged from this mostly Jewish nation but there is an obvious preference for all the foods of the Middle East. Legumes, lamb, fish, and chicken, seeds and nuts, oils, potatoes, tomatoes, eggplant, and eggs are popular. Flat breads share place with raised ones of rye, white, and pumpernickel. Citrus are favorites among the many different fruits consumed, and fresh and dried dates and figs are well liked.

While not all Israelis do so, many observe the rules of Kashruth or keeping kosher. Many other Jews around the world do likewise. This religious maintenance stems from biblical sayings in Leviticus. It translates to an absolute separation of meat and dairy products at meals. Dishes, flatware, utensils, cookware, even kitchen towels may not be mixed and those observing Kashruth require two sets of each of these. Some foods such as grains, fruits, and vegetables are neither meat nor dairy. They can be served with either, such foods that can be used at meat or dairy meals are called "parve" or "pareve".

Observant Jews, like Muslims, do not eat pork or shellfish. Their rituals require that four legged animals have cloven hoofs and chew their cud, that fish have fins and scales, and that no animal eaten be a scavenger. Additionally, meat must be ritually slaughtered in the presence of someone authorized to observe its being done in an approved and humane manner. After slaughter, meat must be salted or soaked to remove the blood.

Commercially, in this country and in others, acceptably prepared and packaged products that meet these religious dietary prescriptions have a 'K' in a circle if they are kosher and/or a 'U' in a circle if they are acceptable to the Union of Orthodox Rabbis. The latter is important to those who are orthodox observers; their food proscriptions cannot be violated. Two other groups, conservative and reform, may use either of these designated products. Background materials on foods and holidays are available in items under Middle Eastern and Mixed Ethnic References.

8.9   Overall

The nutritional strengths and weaknesses in this region are as diverse as the peoples of the Mediterranean. Research indicates that in Iran, 70 to 90% of the caloric intake is provided by the consumption of breads, with a very low intake of animal protein. Fruits are varied, and many of the population exhibit some riboflavin, vitamin A, vitamin D, and even a few ascorbic acid deficiencies. Upon immigration to the United States, cheilsis, hyperkeratosis, and dental disease incidence drops markedly. Immigrants from Iraq have a history of unusually low milk consumption associated with lactose intolerance and the subsequant reduction of intake of related nutrients and protein.

For Greeks, protein levels are adequate, significant deficiencies not obvious, but mineral intake is below the RDA's for iron and calcium both before and after immigration.

Italian immigrants and those in the United States for many years have high levels of obesity and excessive intake of saturated fats. Cholesterol levels and triglyceride values show differences among age groups, regional heritage, and economic level and for some the calcium and riboflavin intakes are marginal.

Turkish immigrants demonstrate a high incidence of iron and zinc malabsorption and Israelis a high prevalence of diabetes. Many of both of these populations are obese.

The Middle Eastern References provide more details. One can see by the limited number of items that more research needs to be done on these cultures.

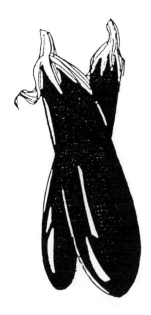

8.10   Middle Eastern References

8.10.1   Mixed Middle Eastern

The following articles pertain to Arab, Italian, Greek, Turkish, and other Middle Eastern food habits and related nutritional concerns. For convenience and because many of the concerns are religious, not just regional, Jewish, Israeli, and/or kosher references are grouped together at the end of this section.

Artigas, G.J.M., Faure, M.R.A., and A, Ballesta. "Gastrin response and local eating habits: Why not spaghetti?" LANCET 1,8166 (1980): 489-490.

Letter to editor questions gastrin response to heavy morning meal. Use of Inmutope kit reveals increases.

Cantoni, M. "Adapting therapeutic diets to the eating patterns of Italian Americans." AMER. J. CLIN. NUTR. 6 (!958): 548-555.

Though three decades since a major wave of Italian immigration to the Unites States, meal patterns, seasonings, holiday foods, and attitude toward illness are still relevant, as are bland, sodium restricted, low fat, and diabetic diet advice.

Darwish, O.A., E.K. Amine, and S.M. Abdalla. "Food habits during pregnancy and lactation in Iraq." FD. NUTR. BULL. 4 (1982): 14-16.

In this study, diets are regionally assessed within Iraq, and show milk, eggs, meat, and chicken eaten more frequently by northern mothers because of their availability there. Fish is eaten more in the south because it is more plentiful in that area. No foods are proscribed during pregnancy but some are encouraged to increase lactation such as milk, butter, fat, dates, wheat flour, and meat. "Hisswo", composed of fat, dates, and flour, is eaten post-partum.

Ferro-Luzzi, A., S. Mobarhan, G. Maiani, C. Scaccini, F. Virgili, and J.T. Knuiman. "Vitamin E status in Italian children subsisting on a Mediterranean diet." HUMAN NUTR.: CLIN. NUTR. 38C (1984): 195-201.

Finds no correlation between serum level of vitamin E and total cholesterol levels. There is a slight correlation between polyunsaturated fatty acid intake and serum vitamin E. Also concludes that this type of diet provides satisfactory vitamin E status.

Ferro-Luzzi, A., P. Strazullo, C. Scaccini, A. Siani, S. Sette, M.A. Mariani, P. Mastranzo, R.M. Dougherty, J.M. Iacano, and M. Mancini. "Changing the Mediterranean diet: Effects on blood lipids." AMER. J. CLIN. NUTR. 40 (1984): 1027-1037.

Investigates adults and finds that individuals with dietary fat changes from 33% to 37% of total energy with animal fats substituted for part of the olive oil show a cholesterol increase of 15% in men, 16% in women; and that men's high density lipoprotein cholesterol stays the same but women's increases 19%.

Fidanza, F. "Changing patterns of food consumption in Italy." J. AMER. DIETET. ASSOC. 77 (1980): 133-137.

Shows increase in protein, fats, and total energy availability over twenty-year period with considerable differences seen in intake and according to regionally.

Fordyce, M.K., G. Cristakis, A. Kafatos, R. Duncan, and J. Cassidy. "Adipose tissue fatty acid consumption of adolescents in a U.S.-Greece cross-cultural study of coronary heart disease risk factors." J. CHRON. DIS. 36 (1983): 481-486.

Using aspiration techniques to obtain adipose tissue, results show 1,5000 U.S. boys aged 8-16 have significantly higher levels of saturated and polyunsaturated levels of fatty acids and significantly lower monounsaturated fatty acids than their Greek counterparts, whether they lived in Greece or in the United States.

Gans, H.J. THE URBAN VILLAGERS, GROUP AND CLASS IN THE LIFE OF ITALIAN AMERICANS. New York: Free Press of Glencoe, 1962.

Describes socioeconomic and ethnic characteristics of Italian Americans in Boston and outlines changes in second generation. Chapter on child rearing also deals with medical care and concerns and attitudes toward compliance. Volume also discusses foods for holidays and daily meals.

Gizelis, G. "Foodways acculturation in the Greek community of Philadelphia. PENN. FOLKLIFE 19 (1970-1971): 9-15.

Looks at adaptations of Greeks and contains much information on diet from taped interview responses of respondents. Includes glossary of Greek food items.

Grivetti, L.E. "Dietary separation of meat and milk, a cultural-geographical inquiry." ECOL. FD. NUTR. 9 (1980): 203-217.

Dietary separation of meat and milk, often considered unique to Judaism, is found in other regions of the world including southwest Asia and some regions in Africa. Moslems do mix meat and milk but there are prohibitions against fish and milk for Berbers in western Egypt. Article discusses these and other related prohibitions.

Gurson, C.T., T. Yuksel, and G. Saner. "Short-term prognosis of protein-calorie malnutrition in Marmara region of Turkey." ENVIR. CHILD HEALTH (April 1976): 59-62.

Researches surviving and deceased urban respondents and finds hemoglobin levels, total plasma protein levels, chronological age factors, weight and height deficits, and hyponatraemia influencing prognosis.

Hershko, C., Y. Gaziel, D. Bar-or, G. Izak, E. Naparstek, N. Grossowicz, N. Kaufman, and A.M. Konijn. "Anemia among Druze children in the Golan Heights." ISRAEL J. MED. SCI. 16 (1980): 384-388.

Finds that none of the 294 anemic children studied have folate deficiency; iron deficiency is cause in all but two. Serum ferratin is less useful diagnostic aid than other less expensive laboratory methods suggested.

Lowenstein, F.W., and D.E. O' Connell. "Health and nutritional status of village boys 6-11 years old in southern Tunisia." J. TROP. PED. ENVIR. HEALTH 2 (1977): 66-72.

Results show number of signs of deficiency increases with age. Genetic differences appear greater than clinical signs.

Mahboubi, E.O., and B. Aramesh. "Epidemiology of esophageal cancer in Iran, with special reference to nutritional and cultural aspects." PREVEN. MED. 9 (1980): 613-621.

Shows that 80% of cases of esophageal cancers are caused by environmental and lifestyle factors and are associated with geography, ethnic background, and gender. They may be caused by different factors in different geographic regions. Dietary concerns include populations with restricted diets or those with overindulgence and high consumption of vitamins, minerals, and trace elements.

May, J.M., in collaboration with I.S. Jarcho. THE ECOLOGY OF MALNUTRITION IN THE FAR AND NEAR EAST. New York: Hafner Publishing Co., 1961.

Second part of this volume concentrates on the Middle East and Egypt, including Iran, Iraq, Saudi Arabia and the Arabian peninsula, Syria, Lebanon, Israel, Turkey, and Egypt. For format and what is included see first May volume under Black American References.

McHenry, S.G. "The Syrian movement into upstate New York." ETHNIC-ITY 6 (1979): 327-345.

Explains some distribution patterns and gives insights and inferences. Shows present day patterns based on historical population movements.

Meleis, A.I. "The Arab American in the health care system." AMER. J. NURS. 81 (1981): 1180-1193.

Discusses perceptions of health care providers as naive and lacking in expertise because the recipients do not expect health care, they expect cure. Care itself comes from other sources. Social characteristics are at the core of Arab beliefs of causes of illness, birth, and death.

Perl, L. RICE, SPICE AND BITTER ORANGES. Cleveland, OH: The World Publishing Co., 1967.

Reviews culture surrounding the cuisine of Mediteranean foods and festivals, customs, traditional foods, and eating habits of the area from prehistory to modern times in Portugal, Spain, Italy, Greece, Turkey, Syria, Lebanon, Israel, and North Africa from Egypt to Morocco.

Sadre, M., and K. Karbasi. "Lactose intolerance in Iran." AMER. J. CLIN. NUTR. 32 (1979): 1948-1961.

Young Iraqis, ages four months to 25 years, are 68% malabsorbers in this population of 105 subjects. Malabsorption increases with age as only 31% of those under three have the problem. Study shows clinical signs of lactose intolerance by 39% of the malabsorbers, and 57% manifest clinical symptoms.

Sakr, A.H. "Dietary regulations and food habits of Muslims." J. AMER. DIETET. ASSOC. 58 (1971): 123-126.

Discusses allowed and forbidden foods and religious observances along with food proscriptions and prescriptions.

Sakr, A.H. "Fasting in Islam." J. AMER. DIETET. ASSOC. 67 (1975): 17-21.

Details significance, demands, proscriptions of day-time eating through the month of Ramadan. Mentions other fasting days, fasting practices, and exemptions from fasting. The latter include the ill, travelers, pregnant and lactating women, women during menstruation, the elderly, insane, and those engaged in very hard labor. For some of those exempted, however, it is necessary to make up fast or give a donation.

Schoenborn, C.A. "Breastfeeding as a contraceptive method among a low income group of Tehrani women." ENVIR. CHILD HEALTH (December 1976): 274-276.

Finds breastfeeding heavily relied on for infant feeding and 54% do so for more than six months. Only 12% express stong faith in its contraceptive effectiveness but 41% believe it is a contraceptive.

Ter-Sarkissian, N., M. Azar, H. Ghavifekr, T. Ferguson, and H. Hedayat. "High phytic acid in Iranian breads." J. AMER. DIETET. ASSOC. 65 (1974): 651-653.

Studies three types of Iranian breads to learn the effect of fermentation time on phytic acid content. Iranian breads are of low extraction flour so long fermentation is unacceptable even though it does markedly reduce phytic acid content. Also discusses man's adaption to high levels of phytic acid.

8.10.2   Jewish, Israeli, and/or Kosher

The articles that follow pertain to Israeli, Jewish, and/or kosher foods. There are a few references above that address Israeli concerns in conjunction with those of other countries, which see.

Bavley, S. LEVELS OF NUTRITION IN ISRAEL. Jerusalem, Israel: Ministry of Education and Culture, 1966.

Describes dietary survey assembled as part of larger family economic expenditure study. Of the 1,610 families, 1,582 are Jewish and all were visited every two to three days to collect data on purchases and other information. Results indicate more families purchase white than dark breads; poultry use is twice that of other meats combined; and purchase of carp is twice that of other fish. There is large consumption of sour cream, but little use of hard cheese; there is low consumption of chocolate, jam, and other sweet foods and large use of fruits and vegetables. The survey also found low consumption of alcoholic drinks, and only a small number of meals were eaten outside the home.

Berkowitz, P., and N.S. Berkowitz. "The Jewish patient in the hospital." AMER. J. NURS. 67 (1967): 2335-2337.

Rabbi and his wife explain religious law as it can affect hospitalized patients.

Burns, E.R., and S. Neubort. "Sodium content of koshered meat." J. AMER. MED. ASSOC. 252 (1984): 2960.

Letter explains koshering of meat by salting and reveals data that kosher meat has at least twice the sodium content of processed meat. For those who must observe this religious prescriptive process, it is recommended to resoak the koshered meat in fresh water for one hour before cooking to prevent sodium overloading by individuals who must restrict sodium intake.

Casner, S. "It's kosher." SCH. FDSERV. J. 32 (1978): 58-59.

Board of Education of City of New York comes up with mixed heritage Jewish-Israeli-Kosher lunch menu that is vegetarian.

Desser, M. "Kosher catering: How & why." CORNELL HOTEL REST. QUART. 20 (1979): 83-91.

Reviews prohibited and permissible foods, ritual slaughter and koshering, separation of food into milk, meat, and pareve categories, kosher equipment and utensil use, and gives a profile of the kosher consumer and kosher catering.

Feitelson, M., and K. Fiedler. "Kosher dietary laws and children's food preferences: Guide to a camp menu." J. AMER. DIETET. ASSOC. 81 (1982): 453-456.

Explains classification of kosher food into its three categories of meat, milk, and pareve. Has glossary of these and other terms. Responses to 308 mailed food preference surveys shows all breakfast items are liked, but prunes, beets, sauerkraut, and chopped liver disliked, so these are not served. Children and camp personnel appreciate use of survey in meal planning for the camp.

Greenberg, R.R. HANDBOOK ON KOSHER FOOD: INFORMATION FOR INSERVICE TRAINING. Riverdale, NY: The author, 1982.

Explains what kosher means, with biblical quotations to explain its origins. Has table of substitutions for converting non-kosher recipe ingredients to acceptable kosher ones. Gives suggested menus for holidays and festival days. Includes product labeling practices, rabbinic supervision, recipes, kosher cuts of meat, acceptable fish, dates of Jewish holidays through 1992, and other related items.

Grivetti, L.E. "Dietary separation of meat and milk, a cultural-geographical inquiry." ECOL. FD. NUTR. 9 (1980): 203-217.

See listing in the preceding section.

Handlin, M.E., and M.S. Layton. LET ME HEAR YOUR VOICE; PORTRAITS OF AGING IMMIGRANT JEWS. Seattle, WA: University of Washington Press, 1983.

Fifty biographical reminiscences, each one page long with photograph. They were taped interviews where elderly expressed feelings about country, problems, and hopes.

Harlap, S., R. Prywes, N.B. Grover, and A.M. Davies. "Maternal, prenatal and infant health in Bedouin and Jews in southern Israel." ISRAELI J. MED. SCI. 13 (1977): 514-528.

Finds mean birth weight of Bedouins born in hospitals about 200 grams lower than that of the Jewish subjects in study of over 13,000 babies. There is little difference in complications of labor or monozygous twinning; Cesarean section rate is more than twice as high among the Jewish mothers and dizygous twinning twice as common among the Bedouins. Patterns of mortality are quite similar in both ethnic groups.

Kaufman, M. "Adapting therapeutic diets to Jewish food customs." AMER. J. CLIN. NUTR. 5 (1957): 676-681.

Explains dietary patterns and typical meal patterns. Modifications in therapeutic diets may be made using exchange lists. There is discussion of holiday concerns. Favorite foods may be included in patient's prescribed diets.

Korff, S.I. "The Jewish dietary code." FD. TECHNOL. 20 (1966): 926-928.

Discusses dietary laws and their interpretations, the meaning of kosher, and the scope and complexity of the laws, kosher meat, kashruth, and food technology.

"Kosher kitchens can provide attractive new revenue." REST. INST. 94 (September 12, 1984): 144+.

Generalized guidelines for kosher kitchens. Gives data where complete information may be obtained. Recipes from Jewish Culinary Art Conference of 1978 for chopped liver and salmon bisque.

May, J.M, with I.S. Jarcho. THE ECOLOGY OF MALNUTRITION IN THE FAR AND NEAR EAST. New York: Hafner Publishing Co., 1961.

See under listing in the preceding section.

Meador, R., and B. Montalbano. "Practical applications of kosher food service in a non-kosher residential health care facility." J. NUTR. ELDERLY 2 (1982): 61-70.

Recommendation is that non-kosher facility not attempt to make a kosher meal but rather obtain one commercially prepared and heat it unopened. Kosher foods in individual containers such as boxes of cereals, yogurt, cottage cheese, and ice cream, and cans of tuna and salmon should be served in their containers. Recommendations for menu writing, policy, and procedures for the diet manual.

Natow, A.B., J.A. Heslin, and B.C. Raven. "Integrating the Jewish dietary laws into a dietetics program." J. AMER. DIETET. ASSOC. 67 (1975): 13-16.

Explains dietary laws or "kashruth", and its therapeutic application. Has list of symbols of approved foods and some food products, and a kosher teaching unit.

Natow, A.B., and J.A. Heslin. "Understanding cultural food practices of elderly observant Jews." J. NUTR. ELDERLY 2 (1982): 49-60.

Includes dietary laws for maintaining kosher food practices, how these practices can be modified for various diets such as low sodium, lactose free, etc. Has Hebrew and Gregorian calendars.

Olowacz, L., and B. El-Beheri. "Kreplach, kasha, and knishes." DIABETES 33,1 (1980): 30-32.

Has hospital size recipes with exchange lists.

Palgi, A. "Evaluation of the dietary intake of the Israeli population, 1949-1977." ECOL. FD. NUTR. 9 (1980): 157-165.

All nutrients except calcium are at higher levels than allowances in 1975, with availability of calories increasing 16% 1949 to 1977. Although current dietary supply is close to United States goals, prevalence of heart disease and cancer is high.

Oalgi, A. "Association between dietary changes and mortality rates: Israel 1949 to 1977, a trend-free regression model." AMER. J. CLIN. NUTR. 34 (1981): 1569-1583.

Shows vitamin A is consistently in statistically significant negative association with mortality rates, and total fat consumption in positive association. Ischemic heart disease, hypertensive, and cerebrovascular diseases are in positive association with both plant and animal fats. Diabetes mellitus is in inverse association with average per capita consumption of fruits and vegetables, suggesting that increased carbohydrate consumption may reduce mortality of this disease.

"School lunch kosher style." SCH. FDSERV. J. 34 (1980): 46-47.

For children who do not adhere to the strictest dietary laws but prefer to follow some of them, certain clearances are allowed by the USDA in serving of kosher meals in U.S. schools. A quantity recipe for a krautball hero sandwich as part of a kosher-style lunch within the bounds of the USDA regulations.

Tamir, I., B. Werbin, E. Tanenbaum, R.M. Pyizer, O. Levtow, and D. Heldenberg. "Serum lipid concentration in newborns from various ethnic groups in Israel." ISRAELI J. MED. SCI. 14 (1978): 970-974.

Results suggest that serum cholesterol at birth of limited value, of the 438 newborns studied again at six and eighteen months, only 36 are originally defined as hypercholesterolemic and 28 had normal values by six months. No differences among the five ethnic groups of this study.

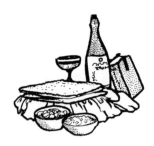

8.11   Middle Eastern Resources for Recipes

Betar, Y. FINEST RECIPES FROM THE MIDDLE EAST. Washington,
  DC: n.p., 1957.

Over 100 recipes, many with uses, origin, and history. Some folkloric stories
and spice and herb lore. Sixteen menu suggestions.

Boni, A. ITALIAN REGIONAL COOKING. New York: Bonanza Books,
  1969.

Translated from the Italian, this edition has recipes divided into sixteen
regions of Italy. Introductory section about the regions precedes the recipe
chapters.

Bugialli, G. CLASSIC TECHNIQUES OF ITALIAN COOKING. New York:
  Simon and Schuster, 1982.

Historical perspectives precede basic ingredient details and recipes by main
ingredient chapters. Considerable cultural information throughout, black and
white photographs of many preparation techniques, and menu suggestions.

Carnacina, L. GREAT ITALIAN COOKING. New York: Abradale Publishers, 1968.

Recipes and many color photographs, both in food category sections.

Casale, A. ITALIAN FAMILY COOKING. New York: Fawcett Columbine,
  1984.

Short introduction, recipes by main ingredient chapters, and many menu
suggestions.

Corey, H. THE ART OF SYRIAN COOKERY. Garden City, NY: Doubleday
  & Company, 1962.

Cultural background, menus, spice and herb glossary, and recipes of Syria
and Lebanon precede the Arabic and English recipe index. Recipes are in main
ingredient chapter divisions. There are also chapters on Lenten foods and menus,
and traditional foods of the Orthodox Catholic Church.

Day, I.F. THE MOROCCAN COOKBOOK. New York: Perigee Book, 1975.

Introductory section provides an understanding of the land and the peoples' customs and religious beliefs. Several variations of classic dishes begin the

recipes, followed by others divided by food category. There are also a chapter on a cook in the Kasbah and a page on Islamic holidays.

Debasque, R. EASTERN MEDITERRANEAN COOKING. New York: Galahad Books, 1973.

Recipes from Greece, Turkey, Israel, Lebanon, and Iran, in main ingredient chapters, follow a short general introduction. Index indicates country of origin of the recipe, many have color photograph.

Grasso, J.C. THE BEST OF SOUTHERN ITALIAN COOKING. Woodbury, NY: Barron's, 1984.

Introduction and each recipe have some background information, recipes are by ingredient categories, and glossary is extensive.

Giobbi, E., and R. Wolff. EAT RIGHT, EAT WELL – THE ITALIAN WAY. New York: Alfred A. Knopf, 1985.

Nutrition information precedes recipe chapters, which are organized by main ingredient. Appendices discuss risk factors, weight and dieting, fatty acid characteristics, nutrient calculations, and menu selection in this book by noted food author and his cardiologist co-author.

Hatton, D. ORIENTAL COOKERY. London: William Collins Sons & Co., 1969.

Chapters on Armenian and Turkish, Arabian, and Jewish cookery, customs, and recipes.

Khalil, N.E. EGYPTIAN CUISINE. Washington, DC: Worldwide Graphics, 1980.

Much cultural information throughout, in introduction, as chapter initiations, and before many of the recipes. The latter are divided by main ingredients in this extensive collection of recipes, most with variations common to Egypt.

Laas, W. CUISINES OF THE EASTERN WORLD. New York: Golden Press, 1967.

Chapter on the Levant kitchen features Turkish recipes, others describe use of spring lamb, Israeli cuisine, breads of the desert, and pastries and coffee.

Machlin, E.S. THE CLASSIC CUISINE OF THE ITALIAN JEWS. New York: Everest House, 1981.

Traditional recipes, menus, and memoir of way of life. Includes holiday celebrations and the popular foods along with their recipes.

Mallos, T. THE COMPLETE MIDDLE EAST COOKBOOK. New York: McGraw-Hill Book Co., 1979.

Introductory section precedes recipes in chapters by country. Included are Greece, Cyprus, Turkey, Armenia, Syria, Lebanon and Jordan, Iraq, the Gulf States, Yemen, Egypt, Iran, Afghanistan, and Israel. Glossary is extensive and includes botanical name and phonetic transliteration of name in countries where used, as well as details of the ingredients.

Nickles, H.G. MIDDLE EASTERN COOKING. New York: Time-Life Books, 1969.

Extensive background material and recipes with emphasis on foods of Greece, Turkey, Arab States, Iran and Iraq, Israel, and Egypt. Roots and current practices are detailed in all the chapters. Recipes appear in this and in the companion spiral bound volume, RECIPES: MIDDLE EASTERN COOKING. Index and glossary give country of origin, recipes do not.

Orga, I. TURKISH COOKING. London: Andre Deutsch, 1958.

View of many aspects of Turkish life precedes the recipes divided by food category.

Rodin, C. A BOOK OF MIDDLE EASTERN FOOD. New York: Vintage Books, 1968.

Introduction includes origins and influences of the cuisines of the region, the traditional table, Muslim dietary laws, and general food information. Recipes are in chapters by main ingredient and most have cultural information of use and custom before the ingredients list. Short bibliography and mail-order source lists are included.

Romagnoli, M., and G.G. Romagnoli. CARNIVALE ITALIANO. Boston, MA: Little, Brown, and Co., 1976.

Meatless cookbook has recipes by meal course chapters.

Root, W. THE BEST OF ITALIAN COOKING. New York: Grosset and Dunlap, 1974.

Some background information followed by recipes in main food category chapters.

Scott, D. RECIPES FOR AN ARABIAN NIGHT. New York: Pantheon
Books, 1983.

Recipes and short introductory materials discuss traditional cooking from
North Africa and the Middle East with Arabic emphasis. Many recipes indicate
country of origin.

Spoerri, D. MYTHOLOGY AND MEATBALLS. Berkeley, CA: Aris Books,
1982.

Travel diary with historical information, cultural items, and recipes.

Wolfert, P. COUSCOUS AND OTHER GOOD FOOD FROM MOROCCO.
New York: Harper & Row, 1973.

Detailed introductory sections on customs and foods precede recipes in chapter divisions by main ingredient. Mail order sources, simple glossary, and short
bibliography.

Wolfert, P. MEDITERRANEAN COOKING. New York: Quadrangle/The
New York Times Book Co., 1977.

Short introductory section precedes recipes from France, Italy, Lebanon,
Egypt, Syria, Israel, North African countries, Turkey, Greece, and Yugoslavia, so
indicated by recipe title, and an index by country. Cultural and food information
thoughout the volume of recipes of home cooking. Mail order source list.

Zane, E. MIDDLE EASTERN COOKERY. San Francisco, CA: 101 Productions, 1974.

Begins with introductory section and each chapter of Israeli, Persian, Turkish, Jordanian, Iraqi, Syrian, Lebanese, and Armenian. Recipes from the north
of Sahara also has a short introduction. Index gives each recipe's country of
origin.

Chapter 9

MIXED ETHNIC REFERENCES AND GENERAL FOOD HABIT INFORMATION

9.1   References

American Dietetic Association, editors. UNDERSTANDING FOOD PAT-
    TERNS IN THE U.S.A. Chicago, IL: American Dietetic Association,
    1969.

Details food habits, preferences and characteristic foods of Chinese, Italian,
Japanese, Jewish, Polish, Puerto Rican, Spanish/Mexican, and South American
cuisines in this 16-page booklet.

Anderson, G.M., and J.M. Alleyne. "Ethnicity, food preferences, and habits
    of consumption as factors in social interaction." CAN. ETHNIC STUD.
    J. 11 (1979): 83-87.

Extensive review of the literature indicates several theories of the importance
of food, the durability of food preferences, food as a factor in ethnic stereotype
formation, and varying definitions of food. Symbolism of ethnic food and drink
explored.

Arfaa, F. "Intestinal parasites among Indo-Chinese refugees and Mexican
    immigrants resettled in Contra Costa County, California." J. FAM.

PRACT. 12 (1981): 223-226.

Stool examinations show 60% of Indochinese refugees and 39% of resettled Mexicans are infected with one or more species of pathogenic protozoa and helminths, primarily hookworm, whipworm, Ascaris, and Giardia lamblia. Rates of infection vary with age and sex, younger persons have greater percent infections.

Armstrong, B., and R. Doll. "Environmental factors and cancer incidence and mortality in different countries, with special reference to dietary practices." INT. J. CANCER 15 (1975): 617-631.

Incidence rates for up to 27 varieties of cancer in 32 countries reveal dietary variables are strongly correlated, particularly meat consumption with cancer of the colon and fat consumption with cancers of the corpus uteri and breast. Discusses limitations and usefulness of the method.

Atkinson, D.R., G. Morten, and D.W. Sue. COUNSELING AMERICAN MINORITIES, A CROSS CULTURAL PERSPECTIVE. Dubuque, IA: C. Brown Co., 1979.

Introduction has overview of how to counsel minorities, three chapters each follow on the American Indian, Asian American, Black, and Latino clients. Book is directed to counselors and mental health practictioners and can sensitize readers to needs of the described populations. References and suggested readings appear after each chapter.

Barer-Stein, T. "Multiculturalism and nutrition counselling." J. CAN. DIETET. ASSOC. 42,2 (1979): 112-116.

Describes Canada's ascent to multiculturalism and the relationship of this and foods and nutrition to the profession of dietetics. Examples of the importance of ethnic diversity rather than its similarity are included for three ethnic groups: Japanese, Russians, and English.

Barer-Stein, T. YOU ARE WHAT YOU EAT. Toronto, Canada: McClelland and Stewart, 1979.

Fifty-two chapters, each on a culture or set of cognate cultures, are included in this extensive volume of ethnocultural food traditions that addresses over 100 cultural groups in North America. Each chapter begins with historical and general background materials, has section on home life, and sections on foods commonly used, meal patterns and eating customs, and special occasions. Foods used are set in four food groups, as well as sweets and snacks, seasonings, and beverages. Source references by chapter appear at book's end and most are books – very few research articles – written by a Registered Dietitian.

Barish, M., and M.M. Mole. MORT'S GUIDE TO FESTIVALS, FEASTS, FAIRS AND FIESTAS. Princeton, NJ: CMG Publishing Co., 1974.

Some ethnic fairs are listed in this volume that is divided by states with sections on Mexico and Canada, as well. Only one or two lines about each festival.

Barth, F., editor. ETHNIC GROUPS AND BOUNDARIES. Boston, MA: Little, Brown and Co., 1969.

Explores the social organization of culture differences by looking at ethnic identity, economic differences, dichotomization, and integration. Three final chapters use Mexican, Pathan, and Laotian groups to show these factors at work. Bibliography appears after all eight chapters. Essays are from a symposium held in Norway in 1967 and illustrate common viewpoints of poly-ethnic organization in different areas.

Bauwens, E.E., editor. THE ANTHROPOLOGY OF HEALTH. Saint Louis, MO: C.V. Mosby Co., 1978.

Reviews clinical and nutritional anthropology, strategies for health care, and perspectives on aging and dying. Volume includes case histories, theoretical perspectives, and original research; each chapter references the latter two. Many ethnic groups are used as illustrations for each of the sections; these can be located through the detailed index.

Benes, P. "Foodways bibliography." FOODWAYS IN THE NORTHEAST. Edited by P. Benes. Boston, MA: Boston University, 1984, pp. 130-139.

Lists primary and secondary source materials on the subjects of diet, food preparation, and cooking in northeast America before the industrial era, and occasional works on Canadian and European studies. These are in four sections: general studies, period recipes and instruction books, archeological and anthropological studies, and architecture, agriculture, and utensils.

Brislin, R.W., W.J. Lonner, and R.M. Thorndike. CROSS-CULTURAL RESEARCH METHODS. New York: John Wiley, 1973.

Concentrates on ways to develop solutions as means of gaining access to cultures, obtaining samples equivalent to respondents in other studies for comparative purposes, writing meaningful questions and translating them properly to assure meaning equivalence across cultures, using known tools of research, interviewing without hostile biases against the interviewees, and gives reasons for data acquisition that are function of the culture and not the researcher's bias.

Brown, L.K., and K. Mussell, editors. ETHNIC AND REGIONAL FOOD-
WAYS IN THE UNITED STATES: THE PERFORMANCE OF ETH-
NIC IDENTITY. Knoxville, TN: University of Tennessee Press, 1984.

Twelve articles by 18 authors of various disciplines are divided into five parts: theoretical considerations, foods as regionalization, new group identities, and food research and the implication of public policy. Specific models used include Vietnamese immigrants, the Mexican tamale, Jewish immigrants, Italian-American experiences, American Hindus, and Florida Seminole Indians.

Brownlee, A.T. COMMUNTIY, CULTURE, AND CARE. Saint Louis, MO:
C.V. Mosby Co., 1978.

This cross-cultural guide for health workers addresses methods for gathering information in various cultures and communities and uses examples from dozens of them as illustrations and/or clarifications. Deals with what to find out, why it is important, and how to go about doing it. Bibliography is in areas and ethnic groupings for easy reference.

Burt, J.F., and A.A. Hertzler. "Parental influence on the child's food preference." J. NUTR. EDUC. 10 (1978): 127-128.

The culture of each family and roles of family members influences food choices. Children of the 46 families and shows that even though mother is the gatekeeper, both parents influence preferences equally, suggesting nutrition education should be geared to all family role models.

Carlson, E., M. Kipps, and J. Thomson. "Influences on the food habits of
some ethnic minorities in the United Kingdom." HUMAN NUTR.: APP.
NUTR. 38A (1984): 85-98.

Current research findings of these and other authors reviewed indicates emphasis on the original culture's food habits. Ethnic groups include Hindu, Islam, and Jain. Descriptions of their food beliefs and nutritional implications of Indian, Irish, Jewish, West Indian, and Chinese cultures. Has many generalizations and specifics about the cultures as well as research findings.

Chen, P.N. "Minority elderly: Continuity-discontinuity of life patterns in
nutrition programs." J. NUTR. ELDERLY 1,1 (1980): 65-75.

Studies 150 Black, Chinese, and Mexican Americans in three nutrition programs and investigates food patterns, health status, social interaction, and program activities and compares them to levels of participation in the program.
There are differences among ethnic groups, with Blacks most satisfied and the
Chinese least satisfied. This is due in part to the fact that the Black elderly are
well assimilated with regard to American food habits and that the other two
groups want to continue to consume same type of food from their country of
origin.

Committee on Food Consumption Patterns. ASSESSING CHANGING FOOD
    CONSUMPTION PATTERNS. Washington, DC: National Academy Press,
    1981.

Volume is intended for Food and Drug Administration and any other agencies, institutions, and individuals monitoring food consumption and nutritional
and health status. Papers on methods of collection and evaluation and nutrition
and health status are a compendium of various authors' views on the available
technology, problems, and practices. Much data on research done serve as illustrative materials for this overview of current practices, but it is difficult to find
ethnic data, as the volume is not indexed.

Coyle, L.P., Jr. THE WORLD ENCYCLOPEDIA OF FOOD. New York:
    Facts On File, 1982.

Alphabetic list of short articles describing how a food item is eaten or drunk
and what it tastes like. Some historical and cultural material. Over 400 illustrations and 53 color plates illustrate the encyclopedia which concludes with a
bibliography and a cross-referenced index.

Croog, S.H. "Ethnic origins, education level, and responses to a health ques-
    tionnaire." HUMAN ORG. 20 (1961): 65-69.

Group of 2,000 army inductees divided by parental origin into Jewish, Italian, Irish, British, and German ethnic groups. Italian and Jewish soldiers have
highest mean number of symptoms and illnesses on the Cornell Medical Index,
perhaps because these ethnic groups verbalize well. In the Italian group, an
inverse association is found between this score and educational level, while no
relationship exists in any of the other groups.

DeVore, S., and T. White. THE APPETITES OF MAN. Garden City, NY:
    Anchor Press/Doubleday, 1978.

Originally published as DINNER'S READY, this volume views what the authors refer to as the "nine healthier societies" of Marquesas, the Tuareg of the Sahara, the Hunzas in the Himalayas, the Gandans of Lake Victoria, the Eskimos, Chinese, Japanese, Mexicans, and healthy people in the United States, most of whom are vegetarians. There are the ones who have escaped degeneration among people who have replaced traditional foods with modern, refined products. This is anthropological, historical, nutritional, cookery and fact and opinion, all supporting the authors' points of view.

Diaz-Duque, O.F. "Overcoming the language barrier. Advice from an interpreter." AMER.J. NURS. 82 (1982): 1380-1385.

Problems concerning the ability of the interpreter, social and intellectual level of the patient, jargon used by either or both, misinterpretation or semantic concerns, unnecessary repetition, anecdotal information use and misuse, and non-verbal behavior, with examples from mostly Hispanic cultures. These highlights bring to the surface many common problems of counseling in another language and culture.

Douglas, M., editor. FOOD IN THE SOCIAL ORDER. New York: Russell Sage Foundation, 1984.

Studies of food and festivities in three American communities, Lakota (Sioux) Indians, Italian Americans, and Blacks and Whites from the same socioeconomic group in a rural Southern community, explore social relations, social change, and social integration in eating patterns and food sharing. Introductory chapter by the editor and final chapter by a computer specialist compare structure of dietary patterns.

Eckstein, E. MENU PLANNING. Westport, CT: Avi Publishing Co., 1973. 2nd edition, 1978.

Section on menu planning with chapters on foodways of Blacks, Chicanos, Native Americans, Puerto Ricans and Cubans, Jews, vegetarians and fruititarians, Central, Eastern, Northern, and Southern European Americans, those in the Middle East, Chinese Americans, Japanese Americans, Polynesians, Indians and other Orientals, and Russian Americans, each with its own bibliography. Introduction to this section alerts dietitians and menu planners to some of the concerns that need to be addressed.

Fant, O.D. "Racial diversity in organizations and its implications for management." PERSONNEL 59 (1982): 60-68.

Recommendations are for an effective workforce of various races, with tips on how to manage and work with people of all groups. Most illustrations are Black-White interactions, but models and concerns can apply to all groups. Discusses recruitment policies and promotional considerations with different value sets.

Fenton, A., and T.M. Owen, editors. FOOD IN PERSPECTIVE. Edinburgh, England: John Donald, Publishers, Ltd., 1981.

The relevance of the study of food to social history is the topic of 33 different contributors. All are papers of the Third International Conference on Ethnological Food Research hosted by the Welsh Folk Museum in 1977. United States, England, Sweden, Ireland, Poland, Austria, Germany, Denmark, Bulgaria, France, Finland, Hungary, Roumania, Greece, and the Netherlands are countries discussed. Each chapter has reference list. Volume has no index for easy accessibility to topics of particular interest in the changes in diet, customs, and traditions of many ethnic groups in different countries, yet much information on these and other topics included.

"Food in many languages." HOSPITALS 38,7 (1964): 165-167.

Albuquerque hospital uses tray aids to teach nutrition to Indians, Mexicans, and other ethnic groups. Diet guides and food lists in Chinese and a number of European languages.

Gelfand, D.E. AGING: THE ETHNIC FACTOR. Boston: Little, Brown and Co., 1982.

Addresses resources and needs of ethnic aged in four major sections. First, concept of and various models suggested; second, examination of sociocultural characteristics; third, the role of mental health, physical health, and social services; and last, a direction for future efforts. Throughout various ethnic groups serve as models; these can be found through the index for individual group study.

Gifft, H.H., M.B. Washbon, and G.G. Harrison. NUTRITION, BEHAVIOR, AND CHANGE. Englewood Cliffs, NJ: Prentice-Hall, 1972.

Addresses nutrition and food behavior through research findings, theory, and empirical knowledge looking at society, culture, and individuals, their food consumption and eating patterns, well-being, and need for nutrition education. References and suggested readings appear after each chapter which provide ethnic materials, though they are not easy to find.

Gordon, J.A., and V. Kilgore. "Planning ethnic menus." HOSPITALS 45,21 (1971): 87-91.

New York hospital considers six ethnic groups in planning their menus: American Blacks, Jews, Puerto Ricans, Italians, Irish, and Chinese. Examples of food habits of each with samples of two breakfasts, lunches, and dinners for each.

Harwood, A., editor. ETHNICITY AND MEDICAL CARE. Cambridge, MA: Harvard University Press, 1981.

Contains chapters on seven ethnic groups, defines who they are, how they came to the United States, their current population and distribution, and suggestions for health and medical care. Includes chapter on culturally appropriate health care for each group.

"How to breast feed your baby." Columbus, OH: Ross Laboratories, n.d.

Handout encourages mothers to breast feed. It and four other counseling aids on breast feeding are available in English and seventeen other languages. Other nutrition, health, dietary, and breast feeding materials also available in many language and media formats.

Jacobson, H.S. SPECIAL DIET FOREIGN PHRASE BOOK. Emmaus, PA: Rodale Press, 1982.

After some general advise of what to do before traveling, and a card to be filled in with personal medical and dietary concerns and tucked into one's wallet, the volume has translations in Spanish, German, French, and Italian of dining out, while following low sodium, diabetic, low fat-low cholesterol, ulcer, and low residue diets. Can be useful not only for travelers, but also for health professionals working with those who are non-English speaking.

James, E.O. "Cultural and religious taboos related to food." PROG. FD. NUTR. SCI. 3 (1979): 67-77.

Reviews taboos, totemism, and dietary regulations in ancient and modern cultures and religions, draws general conclusions, and provides further references.

Jerome, N.W., R.F. Kandel, and G.H. Pelto. NUTRITIONAL ATHROPOLOGY; CONTEMPORARY APPROACHES TO DIET AND CULTURE. Pleasantville, NY: Redgrave Publishing Co., 1980.

First two chapters describe the discipline and its framework. Applications of the model follow from ancient and current perspectives. Models include

Nicaraguan Indians, Mexicans, urban Blacks, and child nutrition in Jamaica. Individually and together chapters are useful, and can provide overall background.

Johnson, H.A. "Other ethnic minorities on the American scene." ETHNIC AMERICAN MINORITIES. Edited by H.A. Johnson. New York: R.R. Bowker Co., 1976, pp. 241-264.

Short introduction is followed by listing of more than 50 annotated films, dozens of film strips, audio and video cassettes, posters, and other graphics on a variety of different immigrant groups.

Keyes, C.F., editor. ETHNIC CHANGE. Seattle, WA: University of Washington Press, 1981.

Contributors address pressing issue of ethnic adaptation and change. Main chapters concentrate on dialectics, direction, speed, and variabilities in ethnic change and ethnic succession. There are also illustrations using Malay, Philippine, Tunisian, Moroccan, Arabian, American Indian, and Asian American data.

Knox, E.G. "Foods and diseases." BRIT. J. PREV. SOC. MED. 31,2 (1977): 71-80.

Chief causes of mortality correlate with main nutrient intakes in 17 countries in Europe, Canada, Japan, and the United States. Findings suggest causal interpretation: alcohol intake and cirrhosis of the liver, cancer of the mouth, and cancer of the larynx; total fat intakes and multiple sclerosis, cancer of the large intestine, and cancer of the breast; and beer and cancer of the rectum. Reviews individual food items and correlations.

Kopito, L.E., and H. Shwachman. "Lead in human scalp hair: Some factors affecting its variability." J. INVES. DEMATOL. 64,5 (1975): 342-348.

Samples children in United States, Japan, Yugoslavia, Iran, and South Africa for significant variables influencing concentrations of lead. Ingestion of lead-containing substances, environmental lead, place of origin, age, and distance of hair from scalp are most significant, sex and nutritional deficiencies least significant.

Lankevich, G.J. ETHNIC AMERICA 1978-1980. London: Oceana Publications, 1981.

This volume updates the chronology series of ETHNIC AMERICA, which can also be consulted. Dozens of ethnic groups have bibliographic materials and history of these minorities are chronological with regard to history, ethnic relations, emigration, and immigration.

Lasry, J.C. "Cross-cultural perspective on mental health and immigrant adaptation." SOC. PSYCH. 12 (1977): 49-55.

Large sample of immigrants' mental health data in Montreal is similar to that of native French Canadians. Cross-cultural comparison shows French-Canadians, North Africans, and Mexicans complain more of psychosomatic troubles than do English speaking Canadians or Americans.

Lieberman, L.S., and V.D. Gardner. SIXTEEN CULTURAL FOOD PATTERNS OF FLORIDA. North Miami, FL: University of Florida, Cooperative Extension Service, 1980.

Black (soul), Seminole Indian, Greek, Orthodox Jewish, Minorcan, Irish, German, Italian, Cuban, Haitian, Puerto Rican, Japanese, Chinese, Vietnamese, and Filipino food habits and practices are followed by foods eaten in each of the basic four food groups, and includes a section on findings, implications, and suggestions for improving or maintaining the diet for best nutritional health. Bibliography for each group, and a general one suggest further readings.

Lowenberg, M.E., E.N. Todhunter, E.D. Wilson, J.R. Savage, and J.L. Lubawski. FOOD AND PEOPLE. New York: John Wiley & Sons, 1979.

This is third edition of text intended for use in general course in foods and nutrition. Historical overview of food patterns, current knowledge, development of nutrition, influences of business, hunger, malnutrition, and government are topics. Each chapter has study questions and references. Culminating reference list and addresses for source materials complete the volume. Index makes accessing various ethnic group illustrations possible, though not always directly.

Manuel, R.C., and M.L. Berk. "A look at similarities and differences in older minority populations." AGING 339 (1983): 21-29.

Reviews population and sex ratios for persons 60 and over and those 65 and over and finds when comparing them, those between 60 and 64 have 2.1% more Hispanics, 2.7% more Asians, 3% more Blacks and 4.7% more Whites. Over half of the older Hispanic population is composed of Mexican Americans; Chinese, Japanese, and Filipinos, in almost equal numbers, make up 80% of the older Asian population. Looking at the 1980 census numbers, 38.1% of Blacks, 30.8% of Hispanics, and 13.6% of White elderly are below the poverty level. Also reviews health status and health practices.

Mason, M. CULTURAL FOOD PATTERNS IN THE UNITED STATES. Chicago, IL: American Dietetic Association, 1976.

This is revised edition of American Dietetic Association item, which see above. Regional and cultural eating practices address Chinese, Italian, Japanese, Jewish, Polish, southern Americans, Spanish and Mexicans, and Puerto Rican groups; information is related to food groups. Includes suggestions for better nutriture.

Mead, M. "Dietary patterns and food habits." J. AMER. DIETET. ASSOC. 19 (1943): 1-5.

Concerns expressed by the executive secretary of the Committee on Food Habits of the National Research Council in 1943 are still relevant today. Offers suggestions, that dietitians can and should provide leadership in educating the public in healthy food habits and balanced meals.

Morin, M.M., L.W. Pickle, and T.J. Mason. "Geographic patterns of ethnic groups in the United States." AMER. J. PUBLIC HEALTH 74 (1984): 133-139.

Eleven maps, based on 1960 census data, show Scandinavian, German, and Russian ethnic groups concentrated in north central regions, Irish, Polish, other East and South European groups clustered predominantly in the northeast. These maps correspond to the atlases of mortality from cancer and other diseases and offer a means of checking if cultural patterns, i.e., dietary practices, match disease patterns.

Murcott, A., editor. THE SOCIOLOGY OF FOOD AND EATING. Aldershot, Hants, England: Gower Publishing Co., 1984.

Four chapters explore food ideologies in depth, two others use limited evidence to do so, and the rest are based on research where food is incidental. All are exploratory essays on the social significance of food and are divided into eating, culture, and social organization; food, health, and generation; and cooking, gender, and household sections. Various ethnic groups provide illustrative material.

Naeye, R. "Causes of fetal and neonatal mortality by race in a selected U.S. population." AMER. J. PUBLIC HEALTH 69 (1979): 857-861.

Other than premature rupture of fetal membranes which occurr more often in Blacks than in Whites, most other disorders are less common in Blacks than

Whites. Other analyses are for Puerto Rican and Oriental infant groups and all are listed for common fetal and neonatal disorders. While significant interracial differences occur, most appear to be non-racial and environmental in origin.

Newman, J.M. "Cultural, religious, and regional food practices of the elderly." J. NUTR. ELDERLY 5,1 (1985): in press.

Overviews fundamental issues and raises questions of what, who, where, and how to help the ethnic elderly. Entire issue is devoted to articles on the ethnic elderly.

Nichter, M., and M. Nichter. AN ANTHROPOLOGICAL APPROACH TO NUTRITION EDUCATION. Newton, MA: International Nutrition Communication Service, 1981.

Volume points out major discrepancy between general recognition that diet is cultural construct and level of cultural sensitivity in nutrition education training materials. Highlights health concerns and suggests ways to improve efforts. It also proposes a community diagnosis and implementation input into regional nutrition planning and offers an extensive bibliography. Many ethnic illustrations throughout in terms of meals, snacks, digestibility, disease, food qualities, life cycle events, etc.

O'Palka, J., J. Mitchell, and R. Martin. "Introducing international students to the American food supply." J. AMER. DIETET. ASSOC. 82 (1983): 531-533.

Pilot study is of one dozen students from four countries, Nigeria, China, Taiwan, and Japan, who learn about American foods and food supply. A two-month follow-up indicates they eat more varied diet with introduction of new foods.

Orque, M.S., B. Bloch, and L.S.A. Monrroy. ETHNIC NURSING CARE. Saint Louis, MO: C.V. Mosby Co., 1981.

A multi-cultural approach includes chapters on Black, Raza/Latina, Filipino, Chinese, Japanese, South Vietnamese, and American Indian patients. Each of these includes history of their immigration, assessment and intervention, communication and language problems, healing and food beliefs, dietary practices including foods in each food group, nutrition concerns, sociological and psychological factors, and biological and physiological concerns. Cross-cultural issues and strategies, research concerns, and references included.

Pangborn, R.M., and C.M. Bruhn. "Concepts of food habits of other ethnic groups." J. NUTR. EDUC. 2 (1971): 106-110.

Surveys more than 110 adults in foodservice, 100 university students, and 65 migrant laborers and finds only casual awareness of foods eaten by people of other cultures. Generally, younger adults mentioned more correct foods and their ethnic association for all six ethnic groups studied, students were least knowledgeable. The six ethnic food groups investigated included Mexican, Chinese, Japanese, Jewish, Black, and American Indian.

Pederson, P., J.G. Draguns, W.J. Lonner, and J.E. Trimble. COUNSELLING ACROSS CULTURES. Honolulu, HI: East-West Center, 1981.

This revised and expanded edition of 1976 volume discusses cultural sensitivities, ethnic and racial barriers, self-awareness, and intercultural psychotherapy. Chapters on Asian Americans, Chicano college students, American Indians, and foreign students detail some methodology and problems. Reference list follows each chapter and last one discusses research and practical considerations.

Pittler, A., and J. Braisted. "Culturally specific food-handling kits." J. NUTR. EDUC. 17 (1985): not paginated.

Discusses culturally specific kits designed for nutrition education of children grades K-6. They address needs of Mexican, Latin American, Chinese, Philippine, and Southeast Asian children and kits are available in several of the languages. They include foods, language, and situations with which the children are most familiar.

"Prologue." WEST. FOLKLORE 40,3 (1981): vii-xii.

Food choice and concepts, assumptions, and ramifications are the topics of this introduction to an entire volume on food habits. Essays that follow include cross-cultural issues, one on a Jewish food, one on a ·Hispanic one, and one on general perspectives in the study of food habits.

Rainey, C. EQUIPPING INTERNATIONAL. Columbia, MO: University of Missouri, Instructional Materials Laboratory, 1978.

Cooking utensils and cooking methods illustrate the variety of food preparation in China, France, and India. Food and kitchen behaviors and instructions for maintaining and using all equipment included.

Revel, J.F. CULTURE AND CUISINE. Garden City, NY: Doubleday & Co., 1982.

Written as a journey through the history of food, the book concentrates on French cuisine but interacts with all other major international food cultures. Index allows referencing food history of other cultures.

Rice, D.P., T.F. Drury, and R.H. Mugge. "Household health interviews and minority health." MED. CARE 18,3 (1980): n.p.

Describes context in which efforts have identified needs in minority health and discusses problem areas which may confound the statistics.

Rice, J.A.S. LEARNING BETTER NUTRITION. Rome, Italy: Food and Agricultural Organization of the United Nations, 1967.

Compendium of what educators should know about food and nutrition and what the public should learn in terms of malnutrition, cultural and psychological influences, social organization, changing food habits, planning applied programs, concepts and content of nutrition education, educational methods, and more. Though more attention is paid to malnutrition than overnutrition, and use is global with third world intent, volume provides excellent background for all, no matter the country.

Robinson, C.H. NORMAL AND THERAPEUTIC NUTRITION. New York: Macmillan, 1982.

This, the sixteenth edition, as well as previous ones, has sections that explore cultural values and food selection practices in general, and in terms of several of the ethnic groups in the United States.

Robson, J.R.K., editor. FOOD, ECOLOGY, AND CULTURE. New York: Gordon and Breach, 1980.

The articles in this volume were first published in ECOLOGY OF FOOD AND NUTRITION, volumes 1 through 5. The ethnic groups discussed are from the Philippines, New Guinea, Tanzania, New Zealand, South Africa, Malaysia, Alaska, and India. The articles discuss diets, food habits, nutritional adequacy, folk medicine, childbirth, food taboos, economic change, religious beliefs, and other aspects of food anthropology and food ecology.

Roman, M. "Ethnic diversity: Older Americans enrich our cities." AGING 339 (1983): 18-20.

Five case studies show how Chinese, Cuban, German and Black elderly contribute to society.

Rux, J.M. "Thoughts on culture, nutrition, and the aged." J. NUTR. EL-
DERLY 1,3/4 (1981): 15-19.

Examines the place of culture and culturally congruent foods in the life of
the institutionally aged. Suggestions made for comparative research on diets.

Salber, E.J., and A.G. Beza. "The health survey and minority health."
MED. CARE 18,3 (1980): n.p.

Emphasizes advantages and disadvantages of National Center for Health interview survey statistics. Examples are from migrant farm workers and urban
Blacks. Points out the need for local surveys to fill minority needs.

Sanjur, D. SOCIAL AND CULTURAL PERSPECTIVES IN NUTRITION.
Englewood Cliffs, NJ: Prentice-Hall, 1982.

Biocultural approach to nutrition, research done, and that which needs to be
done in the field. Divergent dietary patterns are used as illustrative material and
include Americans of many heritages such as Puerto Ricans, Black Americans,
Mexicans, Chinese, Japanese, Vietnamese, people from the Philippines, Hawaii,
and others, not all easily accessed through index, though included under other
headings there. Each chapter has lengthy bibliography.

Seely, S. "Diet and coronary disease: A survey of mortality rates and food
consumption statistics of 24 countries." MED. HYPOTH. 7 (1981): 907-
918.

Finds linear correlation between coronary heart disease mortality rates and
the consumption of unfermented milk proteins with the exception of cheese.
Finland had the highest rates of mortality, Germany half as many, Japan only
one tenth as high, and the milk protein consumption numbers are half and one-
tenth, respectively.

Segall, M.H. CROSS-CULTURAL PSYCHOLOGY. Monterey, CA: Brooks/Cole
Publishing Co., 1979.

Examines human behavior in global perspective and finds it both varied
and orderly. Intended as introduction to the field of cross-cultural psychology;
provides insight into habit formation and enculturation.

Sims, L.S., and L. Light., editors. DIRECTIONS FOR NUTRITION ED-
UCATION RESEARCH – THE PENN STATE CONFERENCES. University Park, PA: Pennsylvania State University, 1980.

Reports on five working conferences sponsored by USDA on eating patterns, nutrition communication, formal nutrition education, community or non formal nutrition education, and evaluation research in nutrition education. Each topic addresses current status, research issues and directions. Provides preconference readings for each of the conferences which can serve as recommendations for the field, and a selected bibliography for those needing more depth.

Spiro, M.E. "The acculturation of American ethnic groups." AMER. AN-
     THRO. 57 (1955): 1240-1252.

Reviews the nature of ethnic research, major studies to date, and what has been learned in terms of acculturation and social mobility, nativism, religion, family, and personality. References cited provide list of major early works on specific ethnic groups.

Spradley, J.P. THE ETHNOGRAPHIC REVIEW. New York: Holt, Rine-
     hart and Winston, 1979.

Volume directed to student of ethnography who wants to do good research. Defines and uses ethnography beyond specific cultures, has good ways to ask questions, gain depth, interviewing techniques, use of informers, and other methodology.

Stern, Z. THE COMPLETE GUIDE TO ETHNIC NEW YORK. New York:
     Saint Martin's Press, 1980.

Though region specific, this volume included for addresses of culturally re-lated facilities that can provide information on religion, land, people, and sources for the 17 ethnic groups in this large melting pot city.

Suchman, E.A. "Sociomedical variations among ethnic groups." AMER. J.
     SOCIOL. 70 (1964): 319-331.

Compares knowledge about disease and attitudes toward medical care and behavior during illness in Puerto Rican, and in Blacks, and four groups of Whites in New York City. Finds the more ethnocentric the group the less knowledge about disease and higher skepticism exhibited toward medical professional com-munity. Puerto Ricans had lowest disease knowledge, followed by Blacks, then Irish.

Thernstrom, S., editor. HARVARD ENCYCLOPEDIA OF AMERICAN
     ETHNIC GROUPS. Cambridge, MA: Harvard University Press, 1980.

Volume is extensive and covers hundreds of American ethnic groups, listed in alphabetical order. Historical background is thorough and statistical material presented, where appropriate. Provides good understanding of each group's migration to this country and its problems since immigration.

Wiglesworth, C.D. "When 'yes' means 'no': The importance of perception in cross-cultural training." TRAIN DEV. J. 37 (1983): 58-69.

Accounts from an area in California are used to illustrate cultural perceptions, misunderstandings, and general problems. Management's need for concerns in these areas are discussed.

Williams, O.D. "Common methods, different populations." CIRCULATION 62, Supplement (1980): 18-23.

Reviews Lipid Research Clinics Program prevalence study and discusses procedures for plasma lipid determination. Study still in progress.

Williams, R.L. "Intrauterine growth curves: Intra- and international comparisons with different ethnic groups in California." PREV. MED. 4 (1975): 163-172.

Suggests poorer levels of maternal nutrition in the United Stated may account for lower position in international comparisons. Results suggest low birth weight resulting from relatively inferior socioeconomic and environmental conditions may explain high infant mortality. Studies White Spanish and non-Spanish, Chinese, Japanese, and Black births.

Wilson, C.S., editor. FOOD – CUSTOM AND NURTURE. AN ANNOTATED BIBLIOGRAPHY ON SOCIOCULTURAL AND BIOCULTURAL ASPECTS OF NUTRITION. Published by J. NUTR. EDUC. as Volume 11, Supplement 1, 1979.

This is second edition of a fifty-page volume that contains references and annotations under a variety of headings. Author index for materials published in the past forty years. Many references from the 1973 edition are maintained. Not complete, but exceptionally valuable, because works recognized as classic take priority over newer items.

Wynar, L.R., and L. Butler. GUIDE TO ETHNIC MUSEUMS, LIBRARIES, AND ARCHIVES IN THE UNITED STATES. Kent, OH: Kent State University School of Library Science, 1978.

Lists 828 locations for more than 80 different ethnic groups, with address and phone number, sponsoring organization, scope, staff, publications, if any, size of collection, and comments about purpose, collection, and services. For some ethnic groups tells of other location sources not listed, i.e., newspaper and organizational archive encyclopedia, etc.

Wretland, A. "Standards for nutritional adequacy of the diet: European and WHO/FAO viewpoints." AMER. J. CLIN. NUTR. 36 (1982): 366-375.

Discusses two types of dietary recommendations and/or standards either recommended or diet actually consumed as percentage of total energy. While ranges are wide, all seem nutritionally acceptable in terms of cultural background, food tradition, and availability. Shows individual nutrient and dietary components.

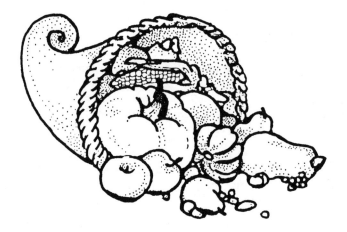

9.2   Selected Resources for Recipes

Cavaiani, M., M. Urbashich, and F. Nielson. SIMPLIFIED QUANTITY
ETHNIC RECIPES. Rochelle Park, NJ: Hayden Book Co., 1980.

Recipes are for 50 portions and are in sections by meal category. Each lists
some dietary information. Some special diet information is included as is a
section of menus from various countries. A few of the recipes can be used for
special diets.

Claiborne, C. THE NEW YORK TIMES INTERNATIONAL COOKBOOK.
New York: Harper & Row, 1971.

Almost one thousand recipes from 45 countries are categorized by country
as are sources for foreign ingredients, which are in broader category groups.

DeRoin, N.R., and T.H. Strenk. "The ethnic cookbook." REST. INST.
April 15 (1983): 17-154.

Discusses Italian, Oriental, and Mexican recipes and foods. Has recipes,
special equipment used, menus, and seasonings with index for the recipes on the
last page.

Gordon, E. CUISINES OF THE WESTERN WORLD. New York: Golden
Press, 1965.

Recipes and cultural materials are divided by use of olive oil, butter and
fat, and corn and beans. Section on the continental kitchen and menus from six
cities are part of this two volume item. This is one of a two volume series, the
other on the Eastern World is by Laas, which see.

Hale, G., and J. Grigson, editors. THE WORLD ATLAS OF FOOD. New
York: Simon & Schuster, 1974.

First quarter of the volume reviews foods by general ingredient item, i.e.,
grains, breads, etc. These chapters provide cross-cultural views of the items
under discussion. The rest of the volume discusses the world of food in 37
country or regional chapters and has a food map, some introductory materials
about the food culture, and then recipes.

Kileen, J., editor. THE WHOLE WORLD COOKBOOK. New York: Charles
Scribner's Sons, 1979.

Includes more than 1,500 recipes from 35 volumes originally published by 101 Productions in chapters divided by food categories. Each of the recipes from the individual ethnic volumes indicated country or area of origin which included India, Hungary, France, Greece, the Middle East, China, and one on the Russian Jew.

Kupfer, J. THE ANTHROPOLOGISTS' COOKBOOK. London: Routledge & Kegan Paul, 1977.

Recipes collected by ethnologists from around the world with comments on the significance of special dishes and means of preparation.

Laas, W. CUISINES OF THE EASTERN WORLD. New York: Golden Press, 1967.

Second of two-volume series, other by Gordon, which see. This one looks east at China, Japan, the world of curry, the levant, and oriental kitchens. Includes recipes and cultural materials.

Marsh, D.B. THE GOOD HOUSEKEEPING INTERNATIONAL COOK-BOOK. New York: Harcourt, Brace & World, 1964.

Originally published for the World's Fair and since reprinted by Avon Books, in paperback, the volume gives recipes for 22 European, four Middle Eastern, 10 Far Eastern, five African, four Caribbean, five Oceanian, four North American, and eight South American countries. One or two sentences precedes almost all recipes and gives background information.

Rozin, E. ETHNIC CUISINE. Lexington, MA: The Stephen Greene Press, 1983.

Introduction includes flavor principles to identify different cuisines. Flavor discussions precede each country or regional chapter; some recipes also have background materials preceding them. Short glossary of foreign ingredients and equipment.

Scott, M.L., and J.D. Scott. A WORLD OF PASTA. New York: McGraw-Hill Book Co., 1978.

More than 200 recipes from all over the globe in food categories with country of origin for each of them.

Von Welanetz, D., and P. Von Welanetz. THE VON WELANETZ GUIDE TO ETHNIC INGREDIENTS. Los Angeles, CA: J.P. Tarcher, 1982.

After an extensive section on herbs, spices, and seasoning blends, the volume looks at the history of each cuisine and then the foods of Africa, Asia, Europe, Latin America, the Middle East, and regional America. Each of these has comprehensive inclusions listed alphabetically of the food items specific to them and detailed descriptions of each. Has recommended ethnic cookbooks, over 150 shopping sources, a recipe index and a general index at the end of this reference volume. The more than 1,000 entries were written with the help of a board of consultants, all experts in their respective fields.

Waldo, M. THE ROUND-THE-WORLD COOKBOOK. New York: Doubleday & Co., 1954.

Recipes are gathered from the 84 countries served by Pan American World Airways and are listed by country. Reprinted many times by Bantam Books.
Also consult:

FOODS OF THE WORLD. A series of 27 volumes on individual countries or regions, published by Time-Life Books, New York.

'ROUND THE WORLD COOKING LIBRARY. A series of 12 volumes on countries or regions, published by Drake Publishers/Garland Books, New York.

Chapter 10

TABLES OF FOOD COMPOSITION

Aagren, G., and R. Gibson. FOOD COMPOSITION TABLE FOR USE IN ETHIOPIA. Stockholm, Sweden: Almqvist & Wiksell, 1969.

Arranged according to food groups, the tables have energy and nutrient data for foods commonly used.

Adams, C.F. NUTRITIVE VALUE OF AMERICAN FOODS IN COMMON UNITS. Washington, DC: USDA, 1975.

This USDA Agriculture Handbook Number 456 has nutrients for 1,500 frequently used foods measured in common household or market amounts. Foods are in alphabetical order, subject index follows.

AMINO-ACID CONTENT OF FOODS AND BIOLOGICAL DATA ON PROTEINS. Rome, Italy: Food and Agricultural Organization of the United Nations, 1975.

This third edition of FAO's Nutritional Studies Number 24 gives amounts of individual amino acids in foods listed alphabetically by food group in the first part of the volume, biological data including NPU, PER, digestibility, etc., in the second part; and an extensive bibliography in part three.

AVERAGE WEIGHT OF A MEASURED CUP OF VARIOUS FOODS. Washington, DC: USDA, 1977.

This Home Economics Research Report Number 41 presents in tabular form, average weight and the standard deviation of a measured cup of a wide number of fresh and prepared foods.

Caribbean Food and Nutrition Institute. FOOD COMPOSITION TABLES FOR USE IN THE ENGLISH-SPEAKING CARIBBEAN. Kingston, Jamaica: University of West Indies, 1974.

Nutrient content of foods are listed alphabetically by food groups. Other tables list amino acids and fatty acids of some foods; the index includes scientific and common names of the food items.

Chatfield, C., compiler. FOOD COMPOSITION TABLES – MINERALS AND VITAMINS – FOR INTERNATIONAL USE. Rome, Italy: Food and Agricultural Organization of the United Nations, 1949.

This FAO Nutritional Studies No. 3 is organized into food groups, has an index of scientific names of the plant foods and an extensive bibliography.

COMPOSITION OF FOODS. Washington, DC: USDA, 1976 to present.

This latest revision of USDA Agriculture Handbook Number 8 is being issued in sections, each with detailed set of tables of nutrient data for a major food group. Each gives water, calorie, protein, total lipid, total carbohydrate, fiber, and ash content, nine minerals, nine vitamins, saturated, monounsaturated, and polyunsaturated fatty acid, cholesterol, and phytosterol content, and individual amino acid content for each food item. Units are in grams, common measures of foods, and pound of food as purchased.

	Loose leaf sections available	Date	No. of items
8-1	Dairy and Egg Products	(1976)	144
8-2	Spices and Herbs	(1977)	43
8-3	Baby Foods	(1978)	217
8-4	Fats and Oils	(1979)	128
8-5	Poultry Products	(1979)	304
8-6	Soups, Sauces, and Gravies	(1980)	214
8-7	Sausage and Luncheon Meats	(1980)	80
8-8	Breakfast Cereals	(1982)	142
8-9	Fruits and Fruit Juices	(1982)	263
8-10	Pork Products	(1983)	186
8-11	Vegetables and Vegetable Products	(1984)	470
8-12	Nut and Seed Products	(1984)	117

de Reguero, L.C., and S.M.R. de Santiago. TABLA DE COMPOSICION DE
ALIMENTOS DE USA CORRIENTE EN PUERTO RICO. San Juan,
Puerto Rico: University of Puerto Rico, 1981.

Lists nutrients of foods alphabetically by food groups. Glossary includes
scientific, Spanish, and English food words.

FOOD COMPOSITION TABLES – UPDATED ANNOTATED BIBLIOG-
RAPHY. Rome, Italy: Nutrition Policy and Program Service of the
United Nations, 1975.

This Nutrition Information Document Series No. 1 is an annotated bibliography of more than 150 published tables that provide information on the
nutritive value of foods. Information listed under reference, background, portion analyzed, nutrients covered, and country.

Food Research and Industry Development Institute. TABLE OF TAIWAN
FOOD COMPOSITION. Hsinchu, Taiwan: FIRDI, 1971.

Nutrient content of foods are in food groups listed alphabetically; they include Chinese, English, and scientific name in the listing.

Franz, M.J. EXCHANGES FOR ALL OCCASIONS. Minneapolis, MN: International Diabetes Center, 1983.

Subtitled "Meeting the Challenge of Diabetes," this volume has expanded exchange list chapters, one on adding fiber to the diet, others on Oriental, Mexican, Italian, Jewish, and camping food exchanges, still others on special occasion
foods. A few recipes are included.

Gopalan, C., B.V. Rama-Sastri, and S.C. Balasubramanian. NUTRITIVE
VALUE OF INDIAN FOODS. Hyderbad, India: National Institute of
Nutrition, 1971.

Tables of energy and nutrients for common Indian foods listed by common English names with scientific name underneath. Recommended dietary
allowances for India and balanced diets and names of Indian foods appear in
Indian languages followed by food index.

Heinz International Research Center. HEINZ NUTRITIONAL DATA. Pitts-
burgh, PA: Heinz Corporation, 1972.

This sixth and last edition to be published has nutrition information and
nutrient content of some foods, composition of Heinz home and institutional
products, and extensive reading list.

Jacobson, M., B.F. Liebman, and G. Moyer. SALT: THE BRAND NAME
    GUIDE TO SODIUM CONTENT. New York: Workman Publishing,
    1983.

Background information on salt, many low sodium recipes, sodium listing
of brand name products by food groups, references, and low sodium cookbooks
appear in this volume from the Center for Science in the Public Interest.

Jardin, C., compiler. LIST OF FOODS USED IN AFRICA. Rome, Italy:
    Nutrition Division of the FAO of the United Nations, 1967.

This Nutrition Information Document Series No.2 is published with the National Institutes of Health's Nutrition Section and has estimated frequency of
consumption of nearly 4,000 foods. English, French, and local names are given
for the food items.

Kraus, B. THE BARBARA KRAUS DICTIONARY OF PROTEIN. New
    York: Harper's Magazine Press, 1975.

Lists calorie and protein content of foods and brand name items.

Kraus, B. THE BARBARA KRAUS GUIDE TO FIBER IN FOOD. New
    York: New American Library, 1975.

Lists fiber content of foods and brand name items.

Kraus, B. DICTIONARY OF CALORIES AND CARBOHYDRATES. New
    York: Grosset & Dunlap, 1973.

This revised edition of CALORIES AND CARBOHYDRATES has more
than 7,500 foods or brand name items with their caloric and carbohydrate
amounts listed, brand name items have company name included.

Kraus, B. DICTIONARY OF SODIUM, FATS, AND CHOLESTEROL. New
    York: Grosset & Dunlap, 1974.

Lists sodium, fat, and cholesterol amounts of foods or brand name items and
sodium content of the water in major cities.

Leung, W.T.W., R.K. Pecot, and B.K. Watt. COMPOSITION OF FOODS
    USED IN FAR EASTERN COUNTRIES. Washington, DC: Bureau of
    Human Nutrition and Home Economics, 1952.

This USDA Handbook Number 32 has nutrient analysis of foods listed alphabetically within food group categories.

Leung, W.T.W., and M. Flores. FOOD COMPOSITION TABLES FOR USE IN LATIN AMERICA. Rome, Italy: Food and Agricultural Organization of the United Nations, 1961.

Has nutrient content of more than 700 foods listed alpabetically by food category. Index includes scientific, English, and local names, and has an extensive bibliography.

Leung, W.T.W., and F.H. Chang. FOOD COMPOSITION TABLE FOR USE IN EAST ASIA. Bethesda, MD: National Institutes of Health, 1972.

Lists vitamin, mineral, and energy amounts of foods commonly used in East Asia. Separate smaller tables on amino acid, fatty acid, some B vitamin, and trace minerals. Index includes scientific and English names; has an extensive bibliography.

Leung, W.T.W., F. Brisson, and C. Jardin. FOOD COMPOSITION TABLE FOR USE IN AFRICA. Rome, Italy: Food and Agriculture Organization of the United Nations, 1968.

Lists nutrient values for over 1,600 food items in plant, animal, and other food groups; these are further subdivided into food categories. English, French, and scientific names in glossary, has extensive bibliography.

Leveille, G.A., M.E. Zabik, and K.J. Morgan. NUTRIENTS IN FOODS. Cambridge, MA: The Nutrition Guild, 1983.

This volume lists 62 factors for over 2,700 foods and brand name items in food group categories. Factors include nutrients, percent U.S. RDA where determined, crude and dietary fiber, 12 amino acids, total fats, monounsaturated, polyunsaturated, and saturated fats, linoleic acid, cholesterol, P/S ratio, preformed vitamin A and RE, beta carotene, total and alpha tocopherols, and 14 trace minerals.

Merrill, A.L., and B.K. Watt. ENERGY VALUE OF FOODS. U.S. Washington, DC: U.S. Agricultural Research Service, 1973.

This USDA Agriculture Handbook No. 74 lists energy data and discusses sources of food energy, digestibility, derivation of calorie factors, and their application, has an extensive bibliography.

Murphey, E.W., B.K. Watt, and R.C. Rizek. "Tables of food composition, availability, uses, and limitations." FD. TECH. 27 (1973): 40-51.

Lists tables of food composition and related literature available from the USDA.

National Institute of Science and Technology. FOOD COMPOSITION TABLE RECOMMENDED FOR USE IN THE PHILIPPINES, third edition. Manila, Philippines: National Institute of Science and Technology of the Philippines, 1968.

Also known as Handbook Number 1, this volume arranges foods alphabetically under general food categories in their national language. Local or common names are given in the glossary.

Pellett, P., and S. Shadarevian. FOOD COMPOSITION TABLES FOR USE IN THE MIDDLE EAST. Beirut: American University of Beirut, 1970.

Nutrients for foods listed alphabetically by food groups, common English and Arabic names are given. Table of scientific, English, Arabic, and Turkish names.

Pennington, J.A.T., and H.N. Church. BOWES AND CHURCH'S FOOD VALUES OF PORTIONS COMMONLY USED. Philadelphia, PA: J.B. Lippincott Co., 1985.

This fourteenth edition gives nutrient content of foods that are listed alphabetically by food categories. Nutrients include calories, fat, water, polyunsaturated fatty acids, cholesterol, saturated fatty acids, protein, carbohydrate, fiber, ten vitamins, and nine minerals. Has large number of fast food items, brand name items, and special dietary foods. Supplementary tables of amino acids, alcoholic beverages, infant formulas, margarines, nine additional minerals, five vitamins; includes caffeine content of some foods and drugs.

Polacci, W., J.S. McHargue, and B.P. Perloff, principal investigators. FOOD COMPOSITION TABLES FOR THE NEAR EAST. London, England: Her Majesty's Stationery Office, 1962.

Revised edition of SRS Number 253, this special report, Series Number 302, gives two minerals, five vitamins, and six other nutrients in foods listed alphabetically by food groups. Glossary of scientific and common English names follows.

Tung, T.C., P.C. Huang, H.C. Li, and H.L. Chen. COMPOSITION OF FOODS USED IN TAIWAN. Taipei, Taiwan: Reprinted from the J. FORMOSAN MED. ASSOC. 60,11 (1961): 973-1005.

Nutrient content of foods listed alphabetically by food group categories.
Foods are written with Chinese, English, and scientific names.

United States Department of Agriculture. GUIDE TO THE SODIUM CON-
TENT OF YOUR FOOD. New York: Dover Publications, 1984.

After short introduction, lists foods alphabetically by food categories and
gives portion size, weight, and sodium content. Section on non-prescription
drugs completes the paperback.

U.S. Interdepartmental Committee on Nutrition for National Defense. FOOD
COMPOSITION TABLE FOR USE IN LATIN AMERICA. Bethesda,
MD: ICNND, 1961.

Lists nutrient data for over 700 foods and has conversion factors for weights
in various countries. Glossary has Spanish, English, and scientific names, and
an extensive bibliography.

Visser, F.R., and J.K. Burrows. COMPOSITION OF NEW ZEALAND
FOODS. Wellington, New Zealand: Applied Chemistry Division of the
New Zealand Department of Scientific and Industrial Research, 1983.

First in what is planned to be a series of volumes, this one indicates composition of sixteen characteristic fruits and vegetables by water, reducing and total
sugar, starch, fiber, protein, fat, energy, eleven minerals, and seven vitamins.
Each of the food items has color photograph, detailed food notes of origin, uses,
and means employed in the analysis.

Watt, B.K., and A.L. Merrill. COMPOSITION OF FOODS. Washington,
DC: United Stated Department of Agriculture, 1963.

This Agriculture Handbook Number 8 is a one volume item with foods listed
alphabetically with their nutrient content in 100 gram and one pound amounts.
It is now superceded by Numbers 8-1 through 8-12. Future volumes will be
released when completed.

Wilford, L., editor. NUTRITIVE VALUE OF CONVENIENCE FOODS.
Hines, IL: West Suburban Dietetic Association, 1982.

Lists portion size, calories, protein, carbohydrate, fat, cholesterol, sodium,
and potassium of hundreds of packaged foods by food category.

Yu, S.M., translator. TABLE OF FOOD COMPOSITION (SHIWU CHENGFEN
BIAO). Beijing (Peking), China: Department of Nutrition of the Chinese
Academy of Medical Sciences, 1981.

Nutrient composition of foods listed by food groups with additional chapters on wild vegetables, amino acid, fatty acid, and nutrients of foods not listed in the main tables. Scientific names of foods and of some wild vegetables at the end of the volume.